THE PICTURE BOOK OF
WILDLIFE

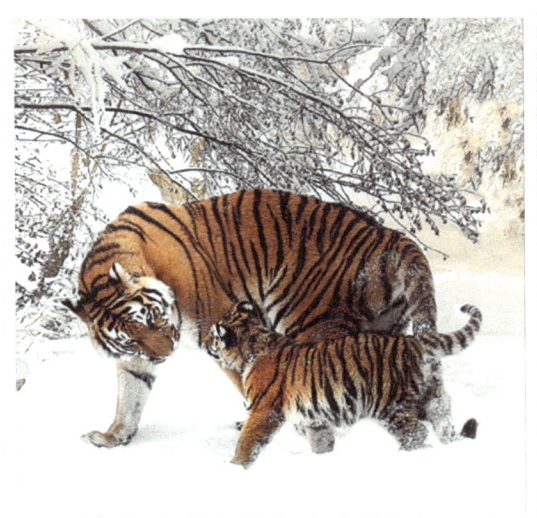

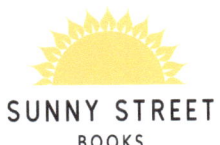

SUNNY STREET
BOOKS

Copyright © 2022 Sunny Street Books
All rights reserved.

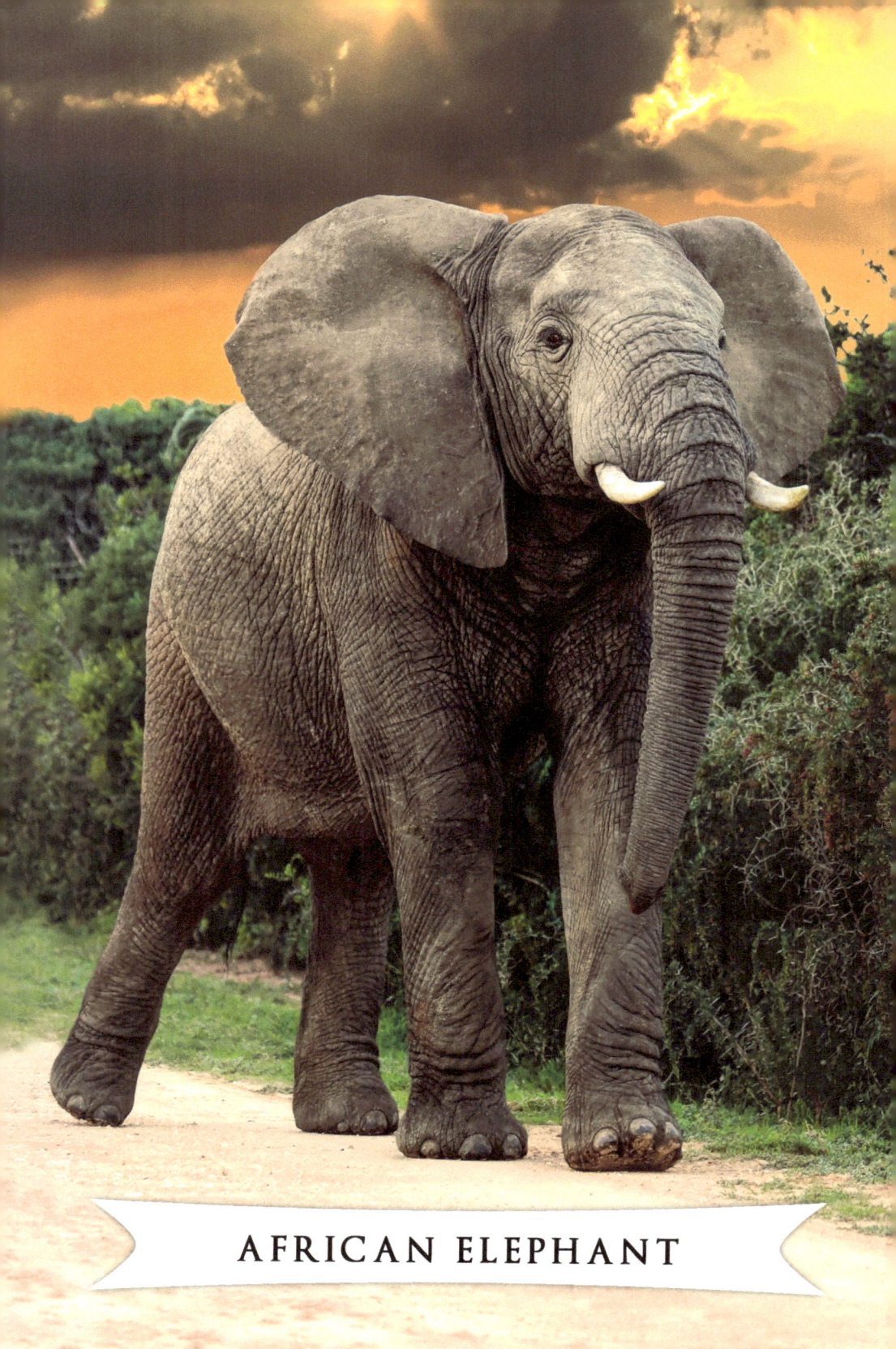

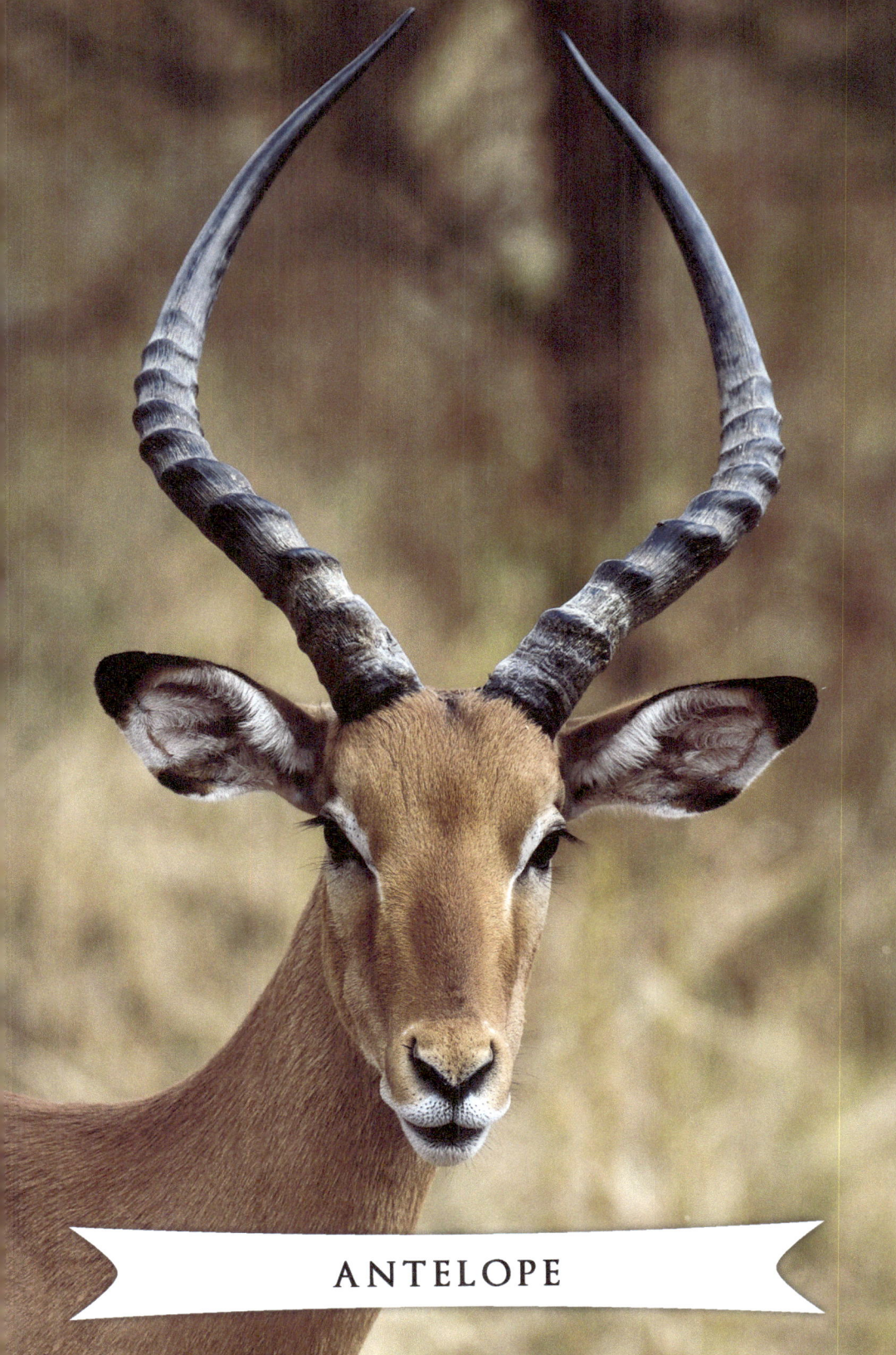

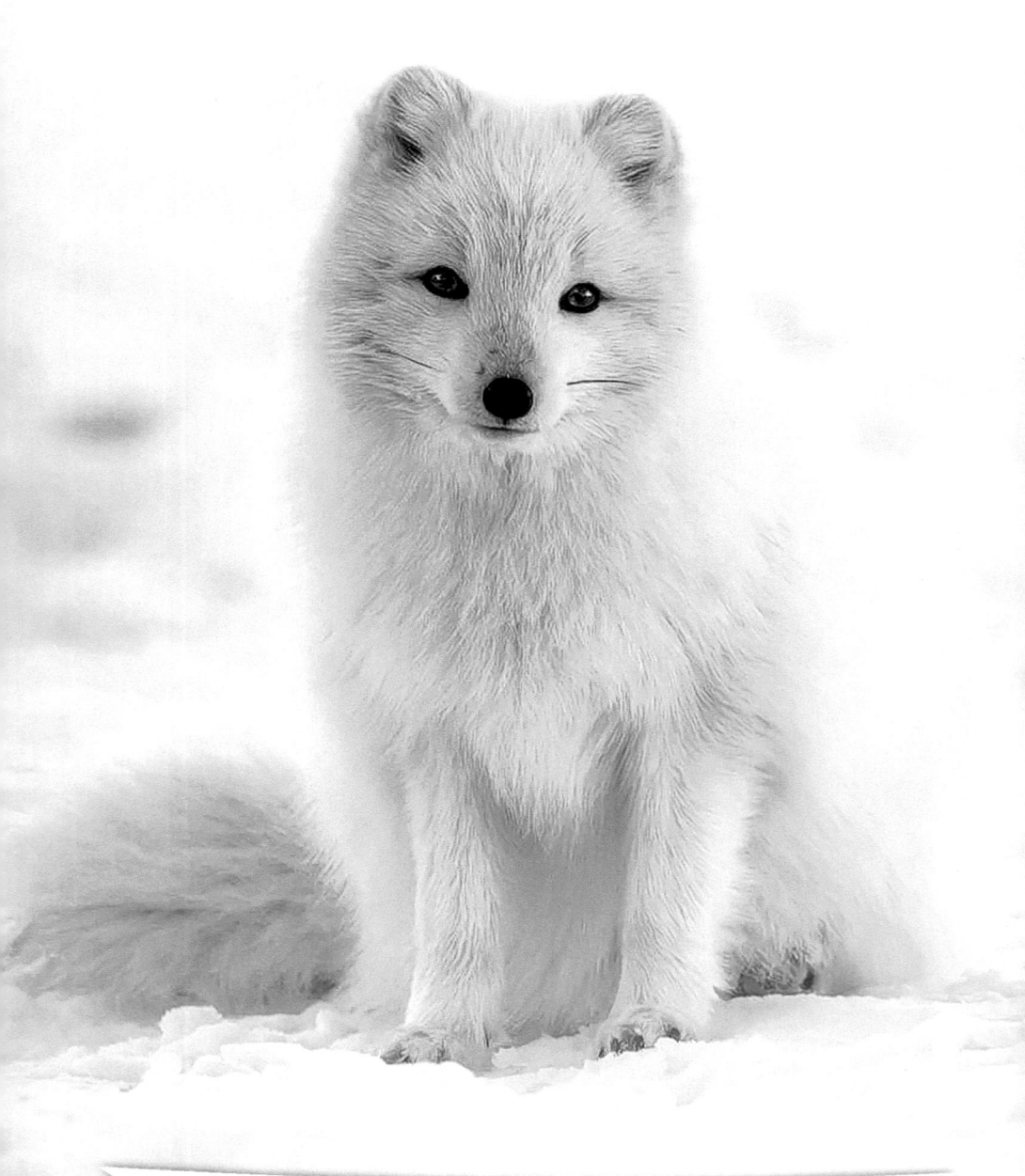

ARCTIC FOX

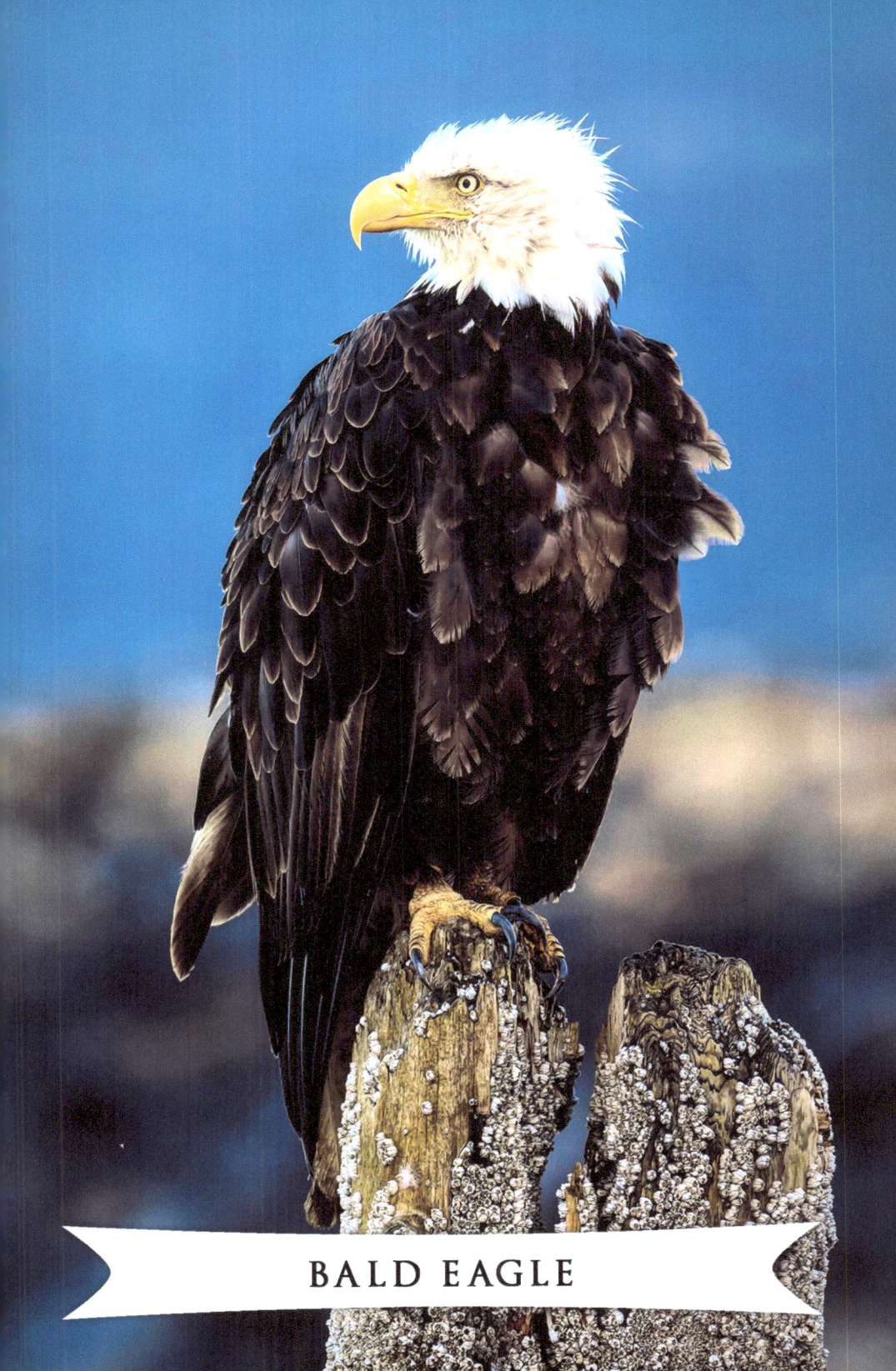

BALD EAGLE

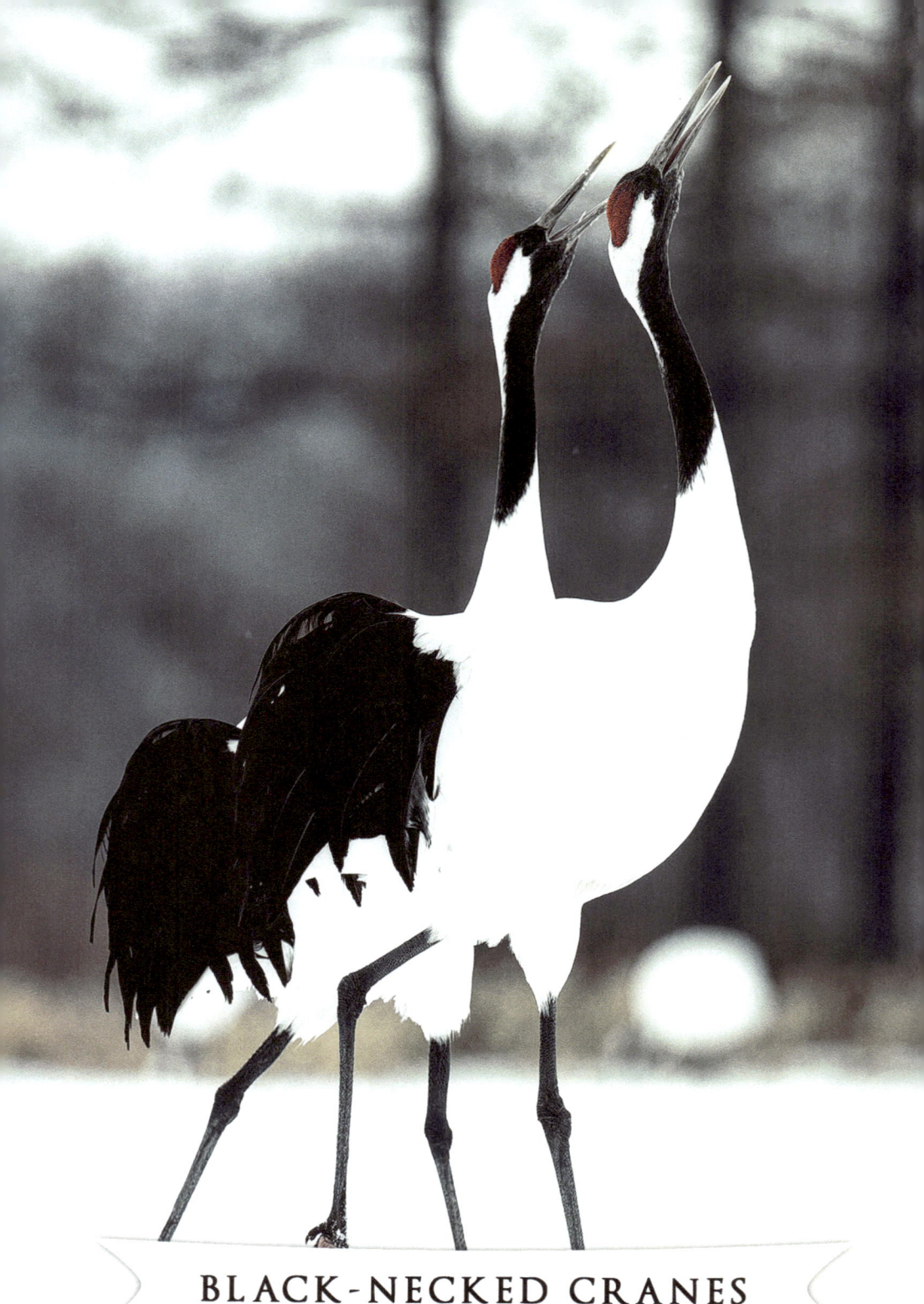
BLACK-NECKED CRANES

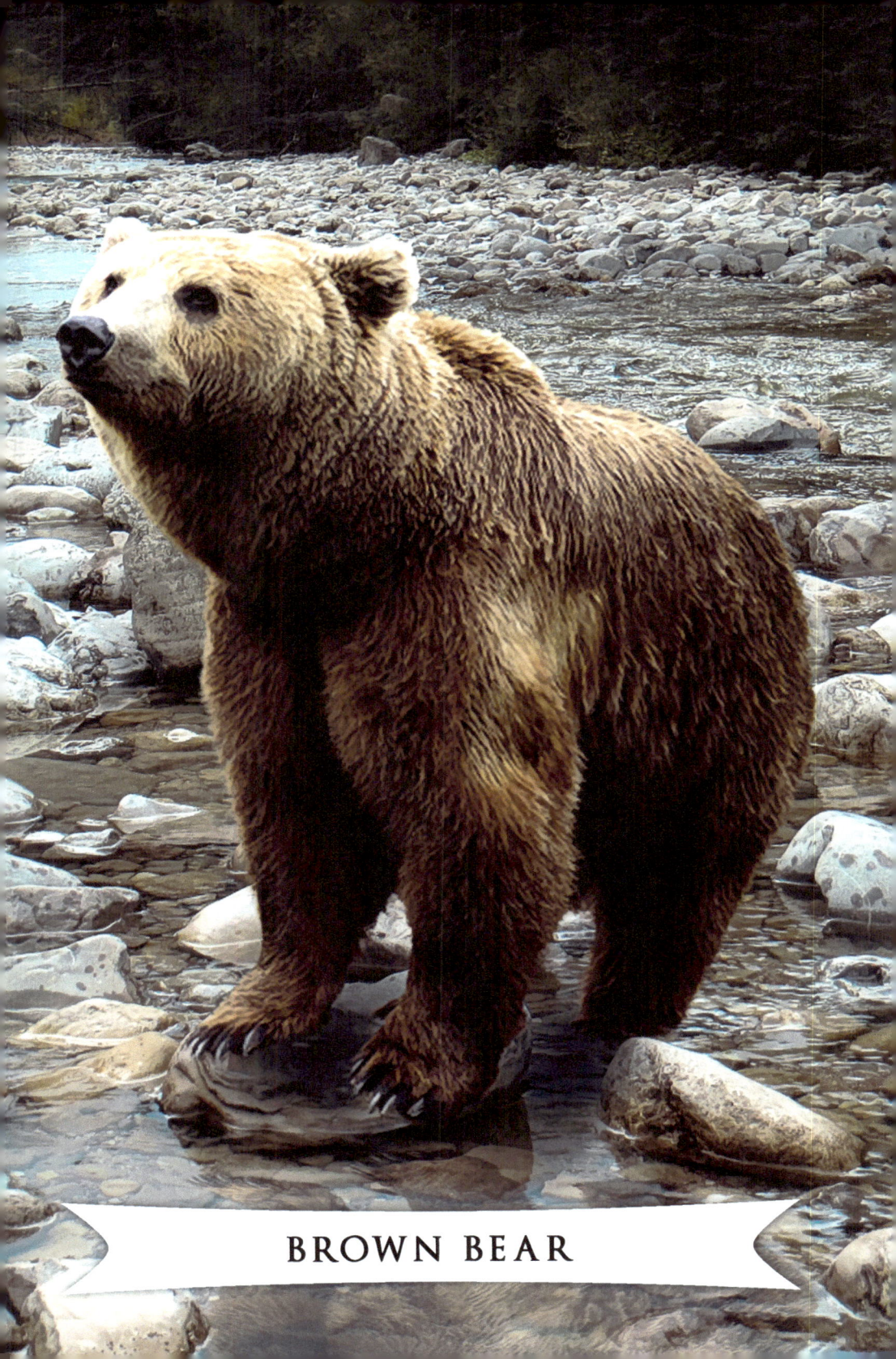
BROWN BEAR

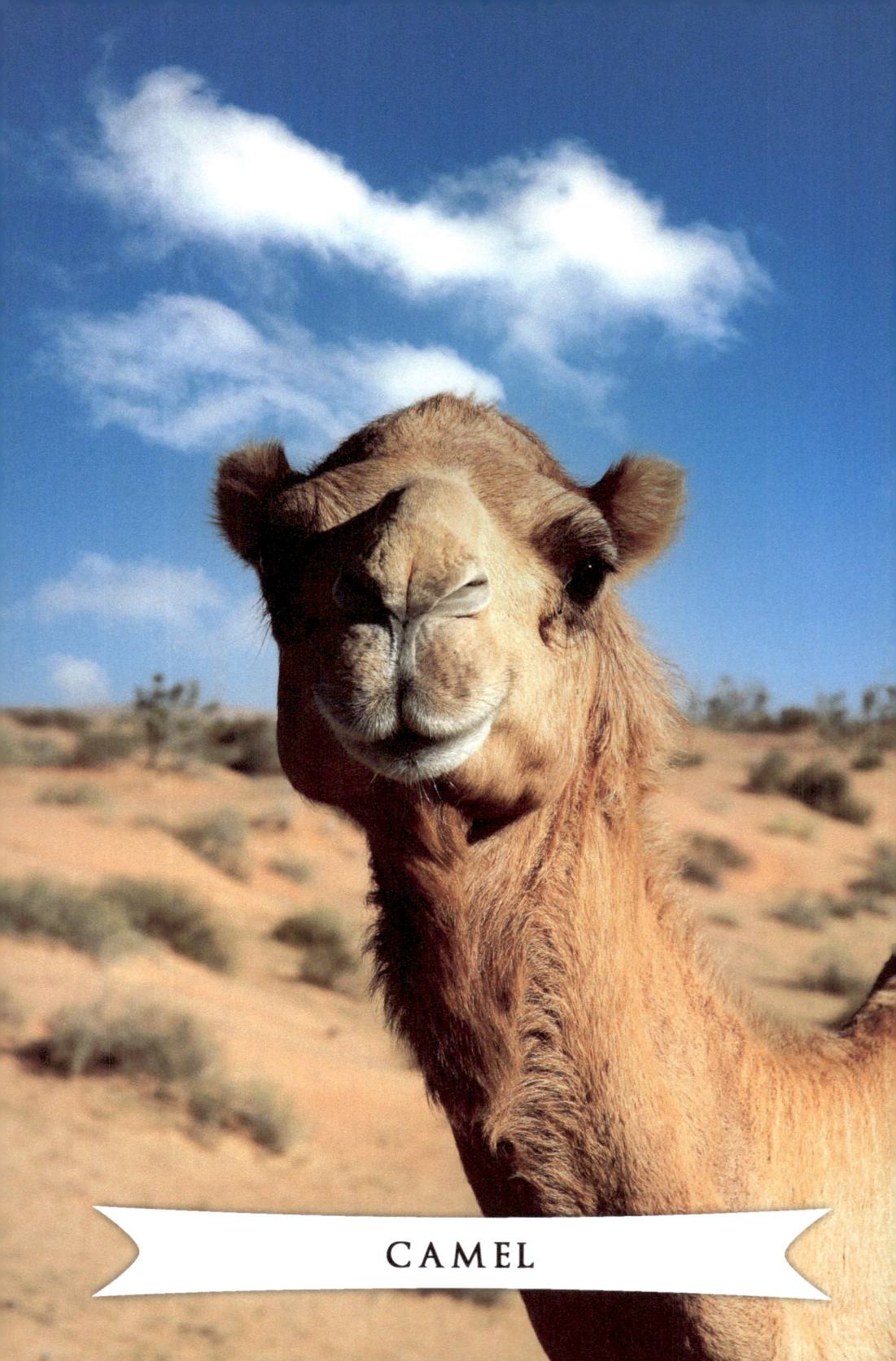
CAMEL

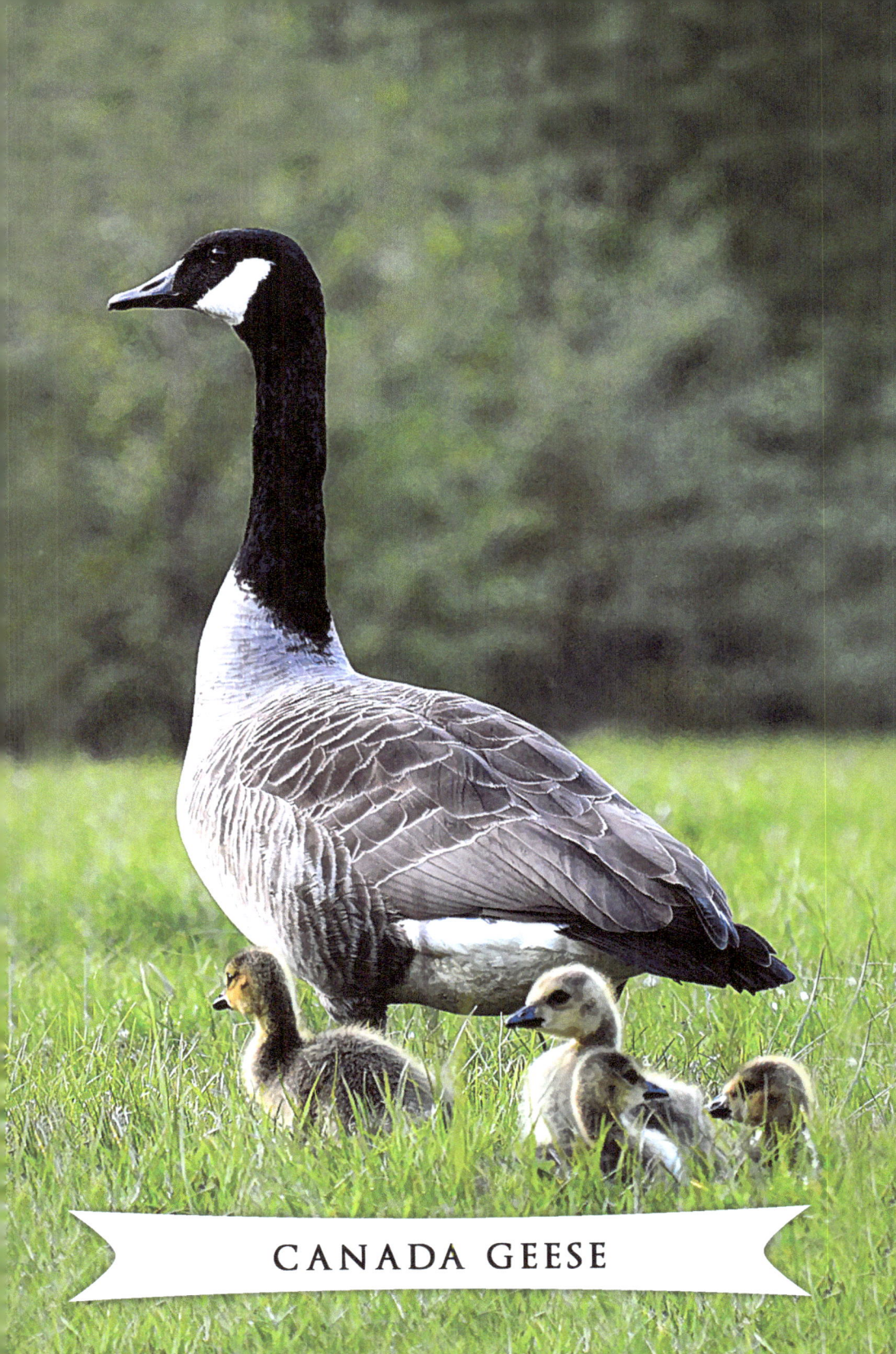
CANADA GEESE

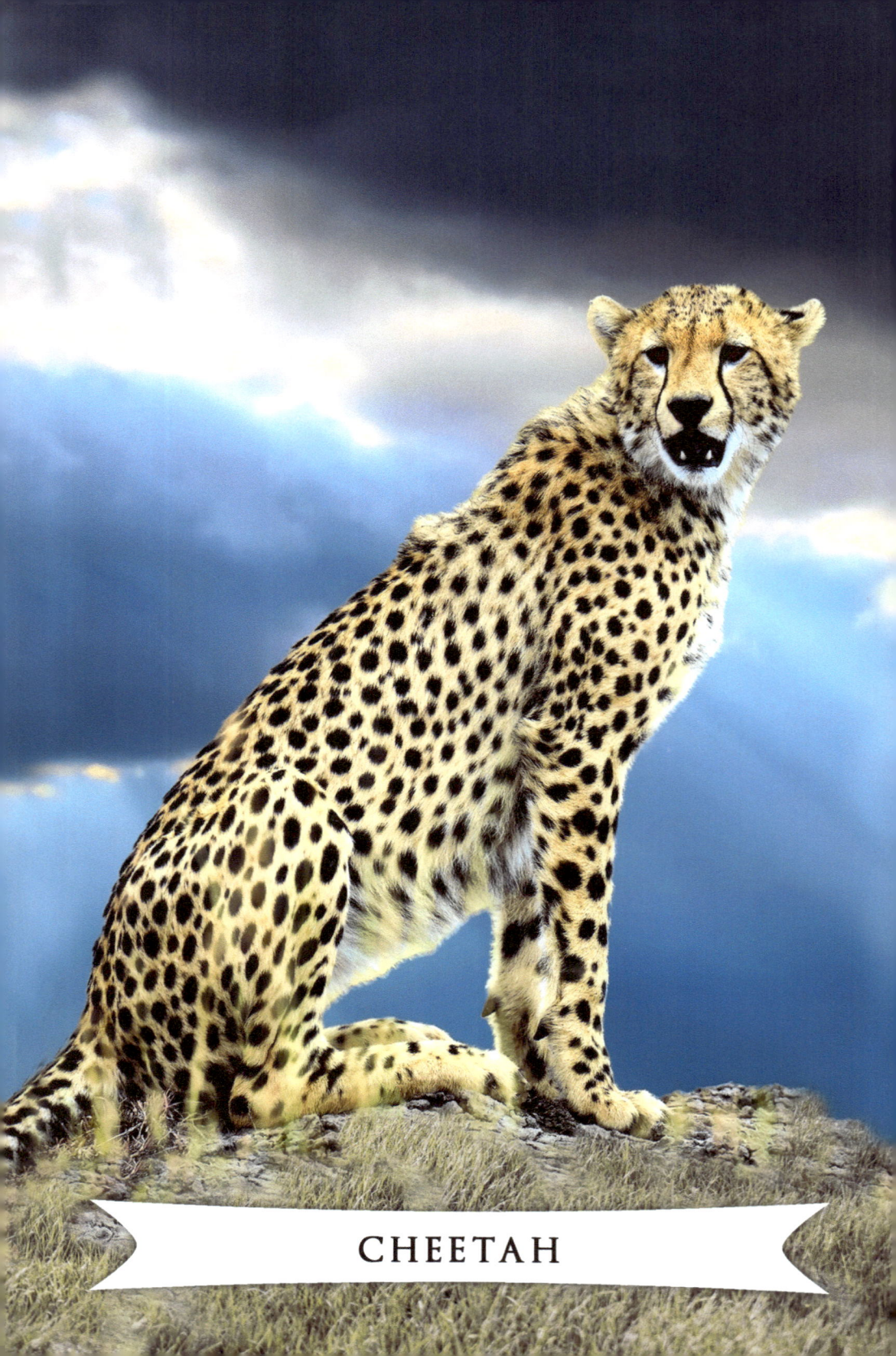

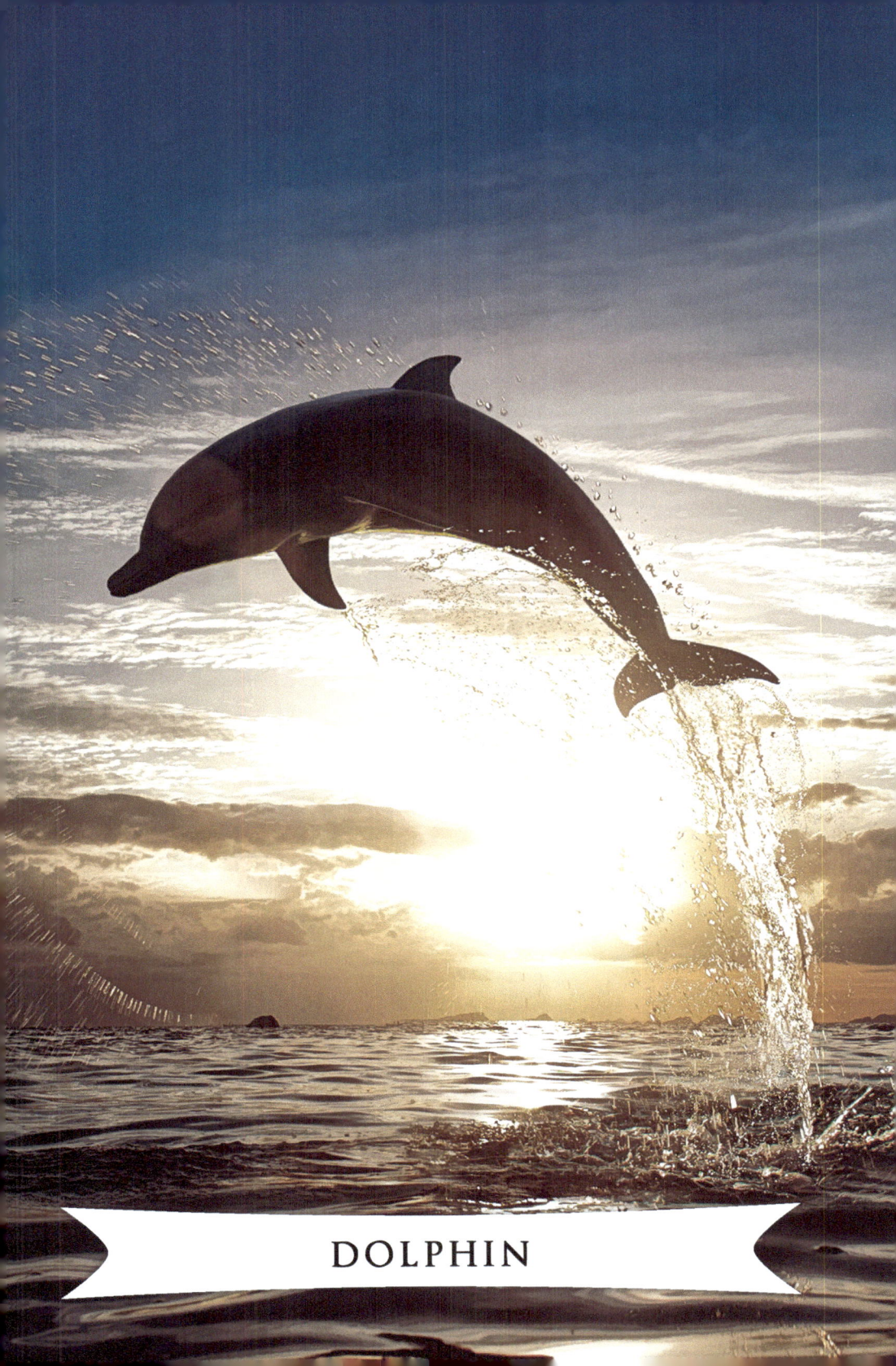

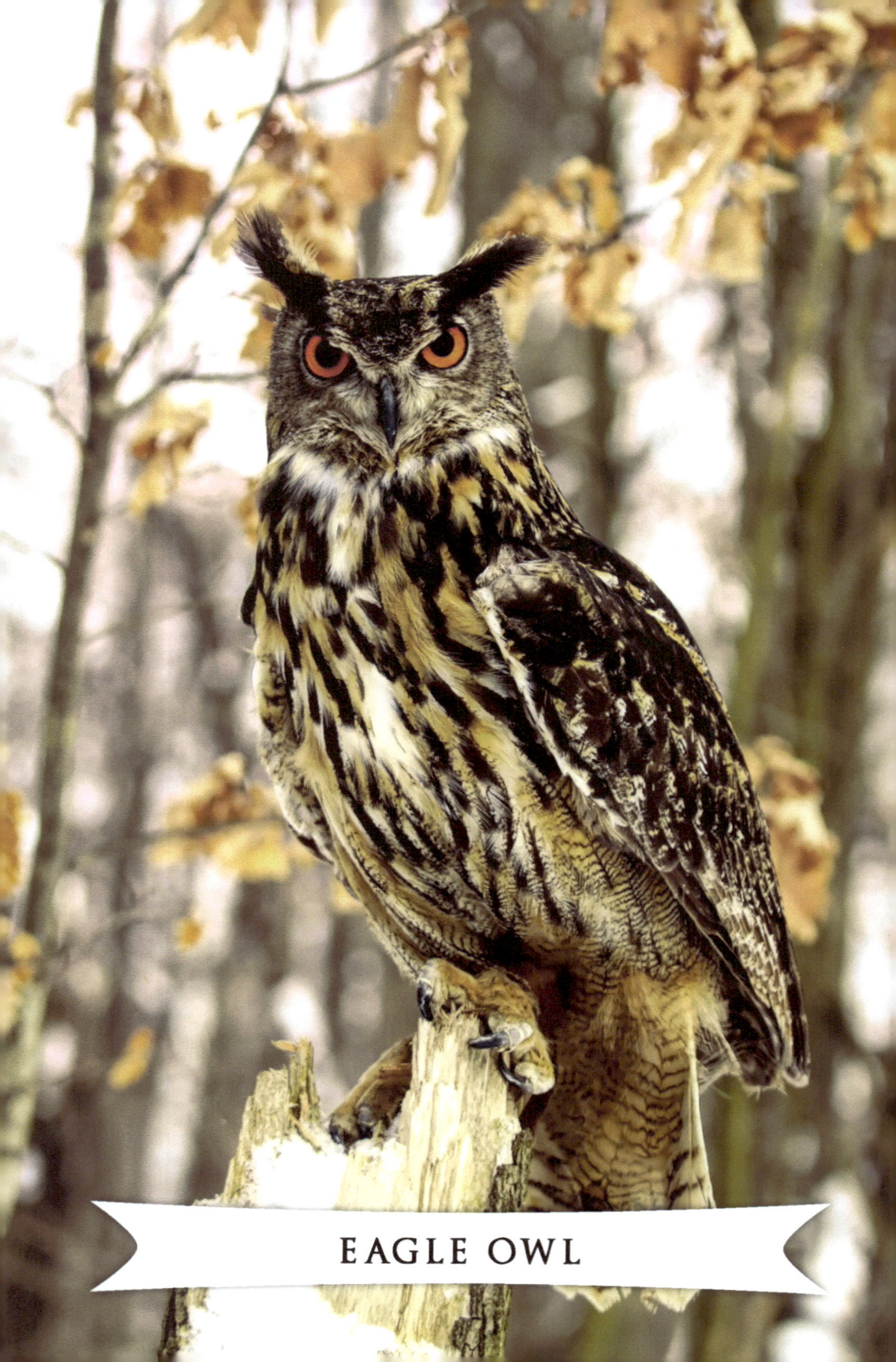

EAGLE OWL

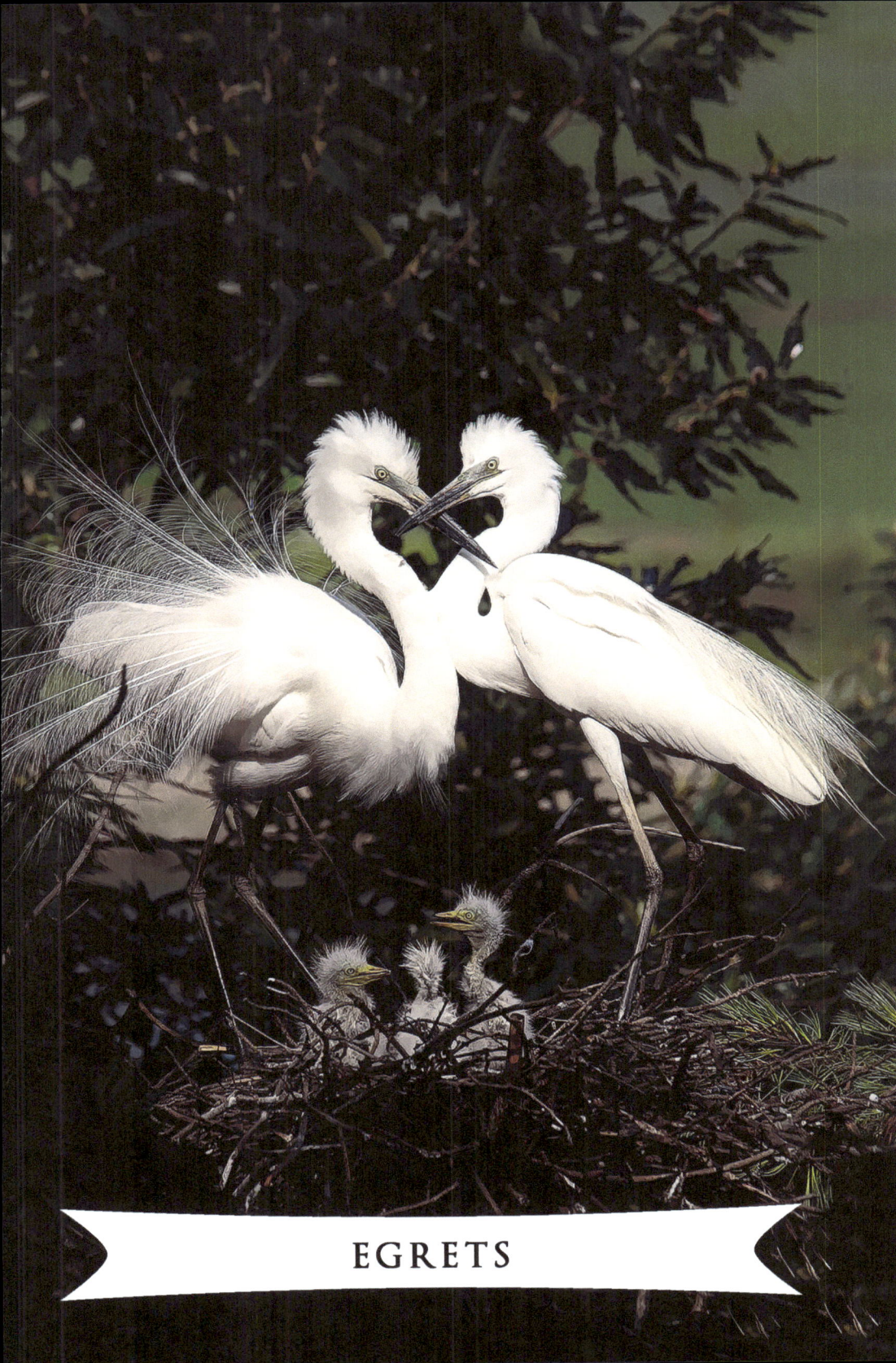

EGRETS

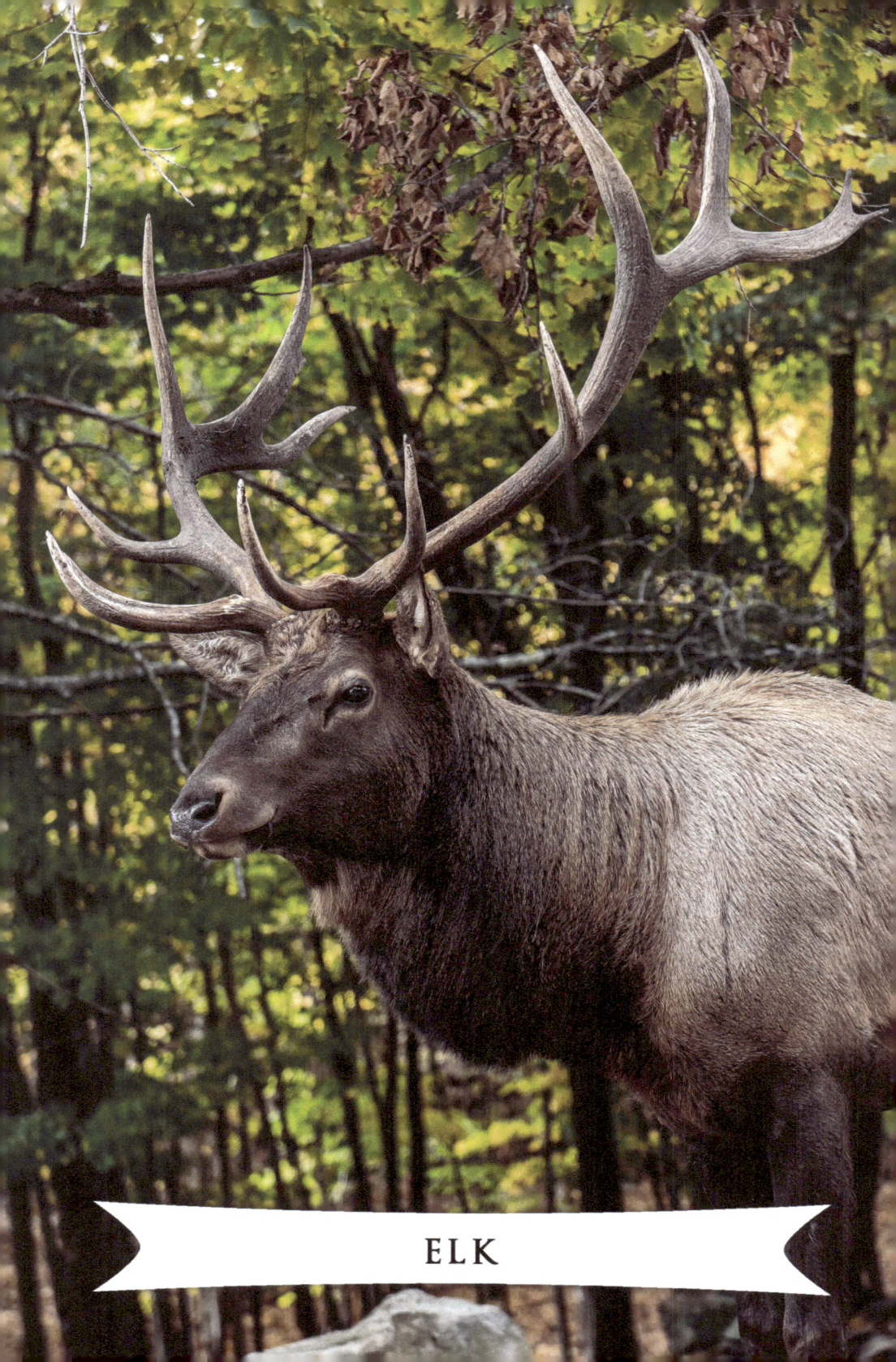

ELK

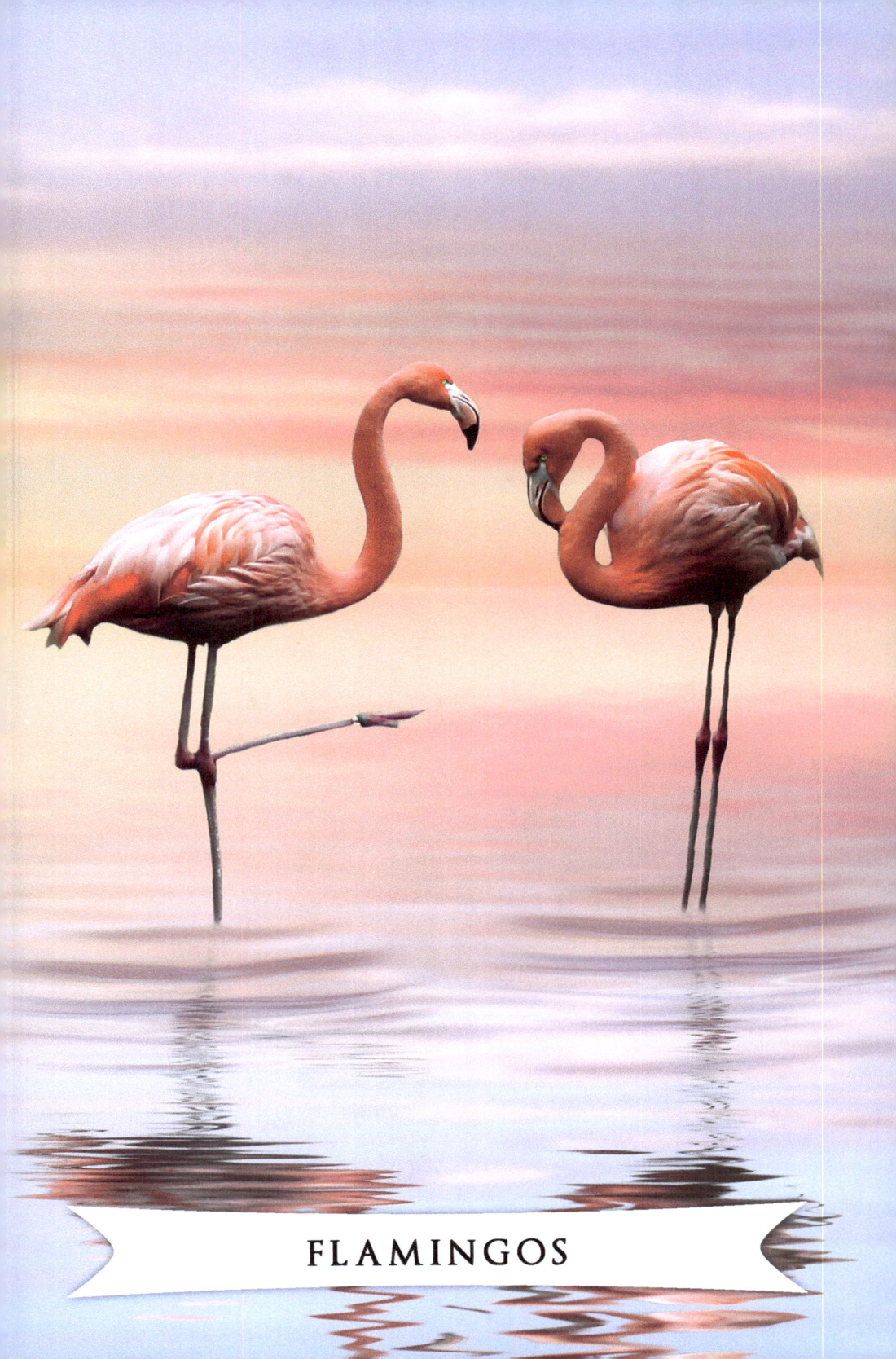

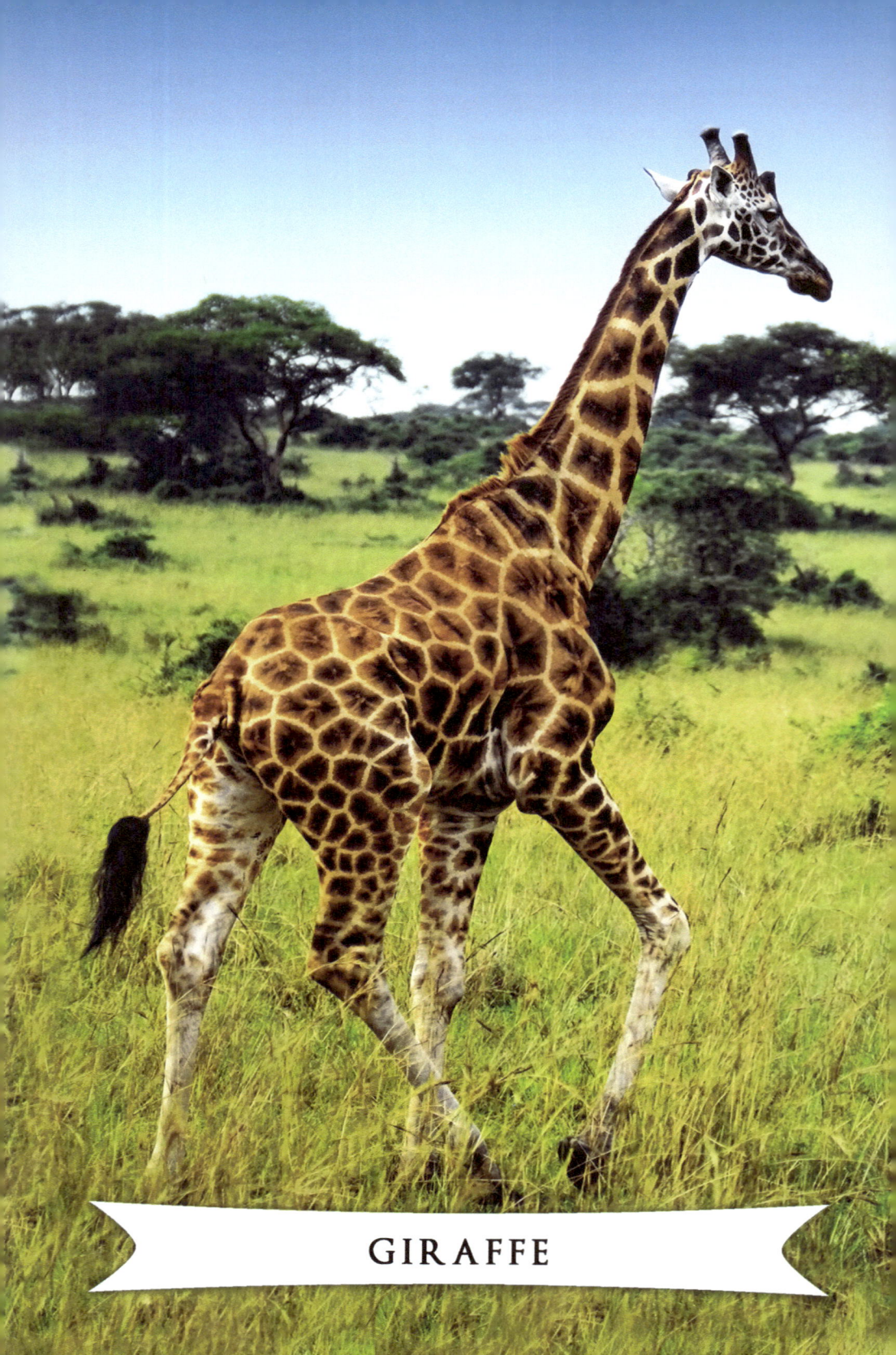
GIRAFFE

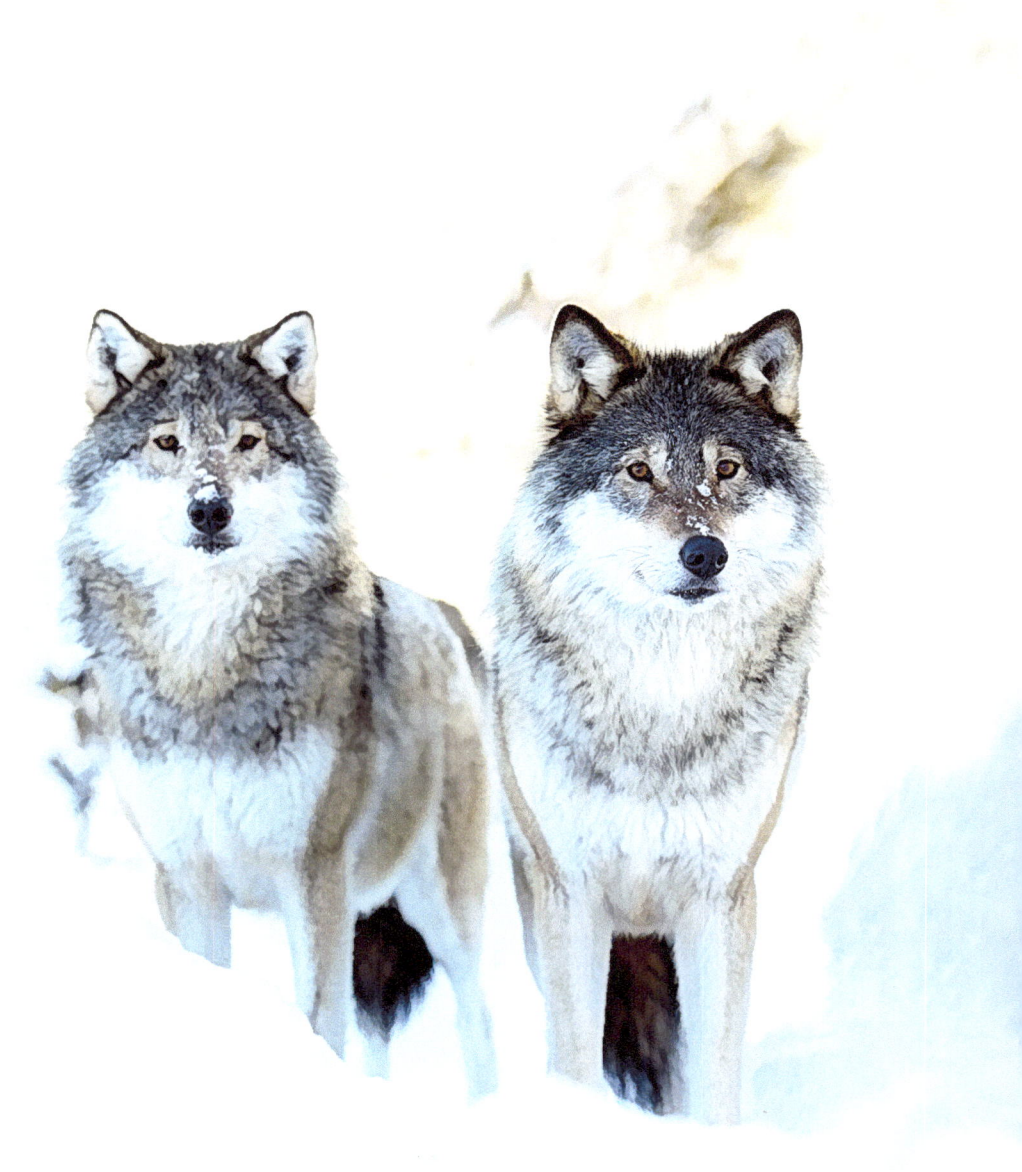

GRAY WOLVES

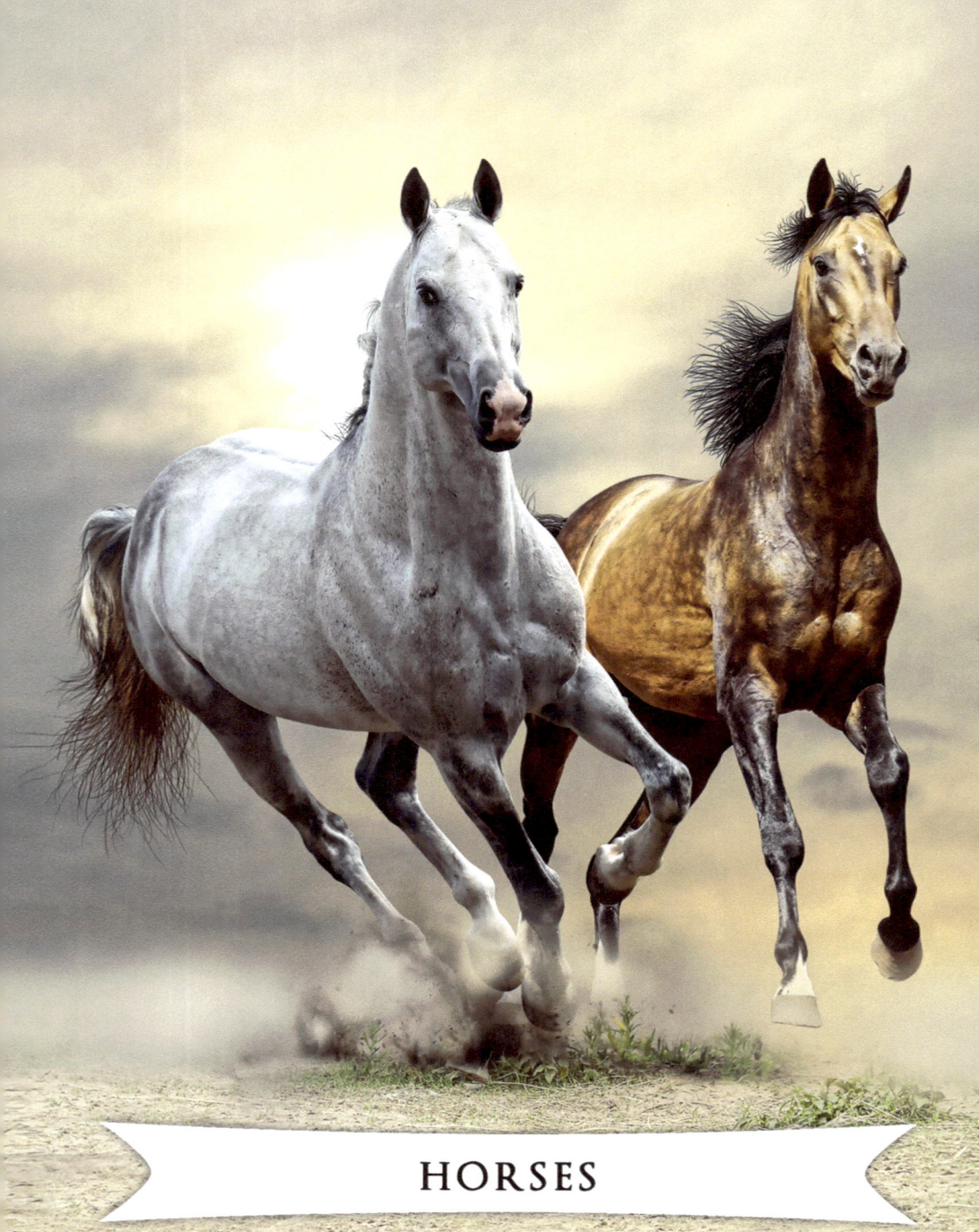

HORSES

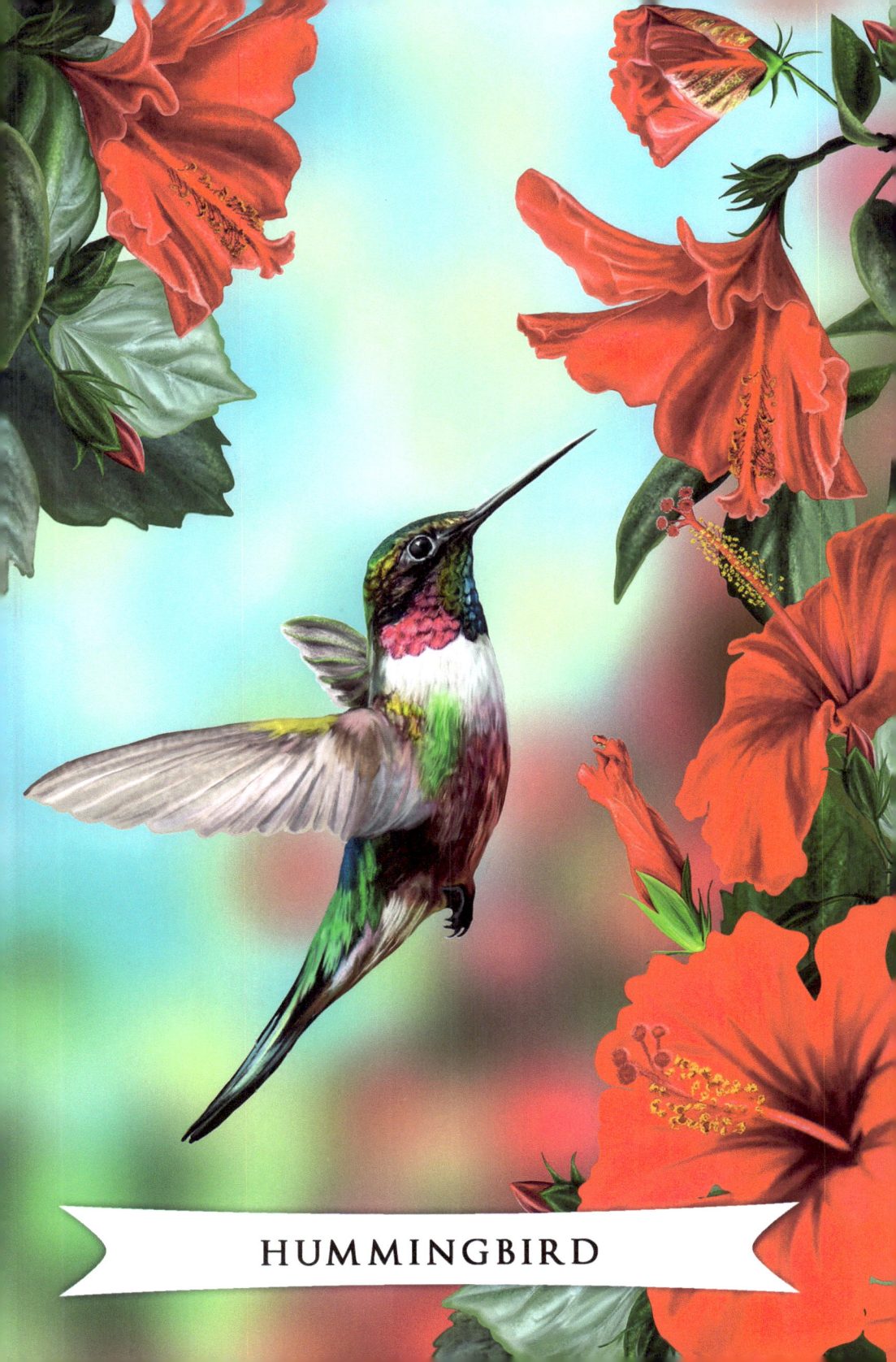

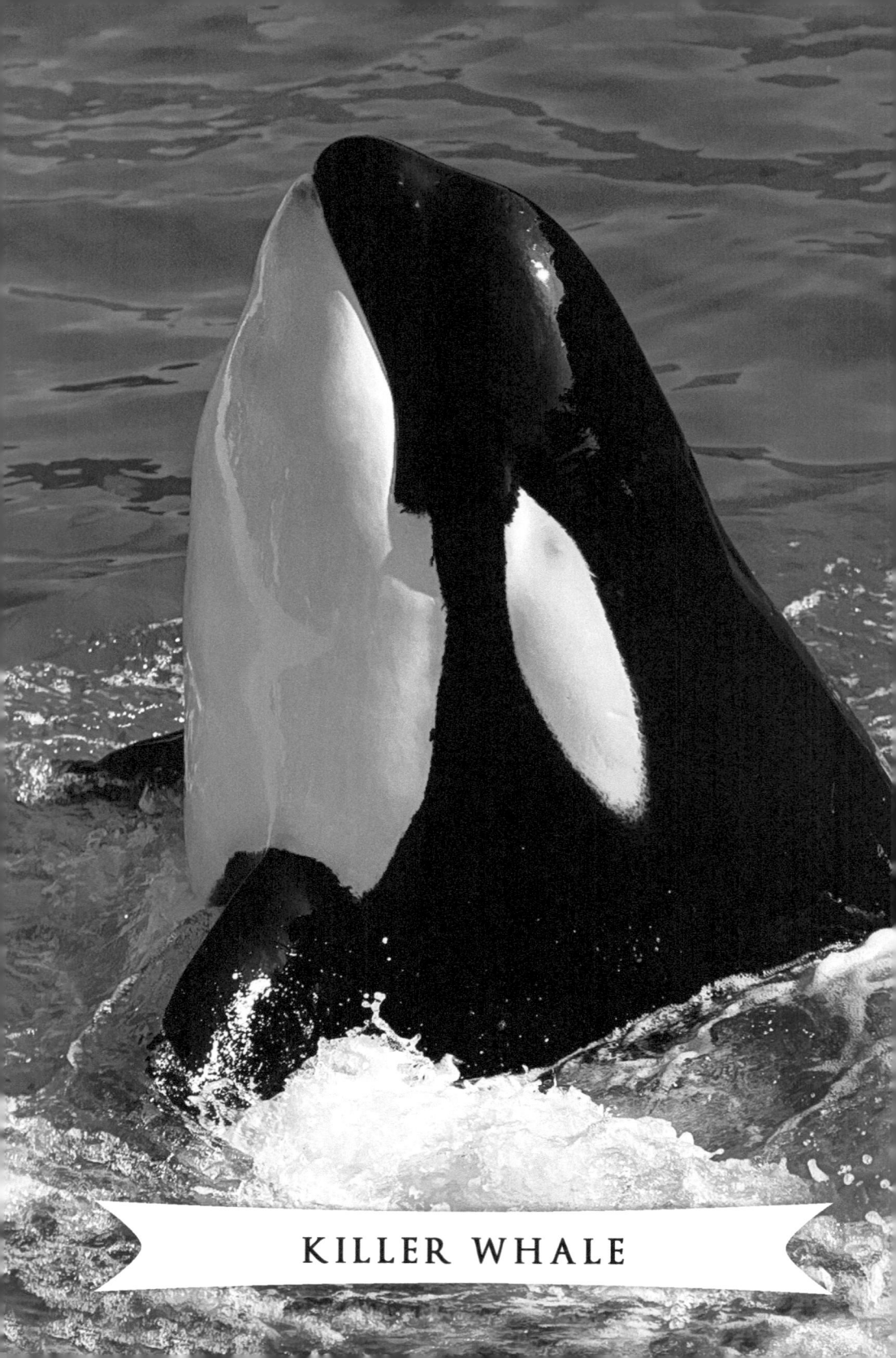
KILLER WHALE

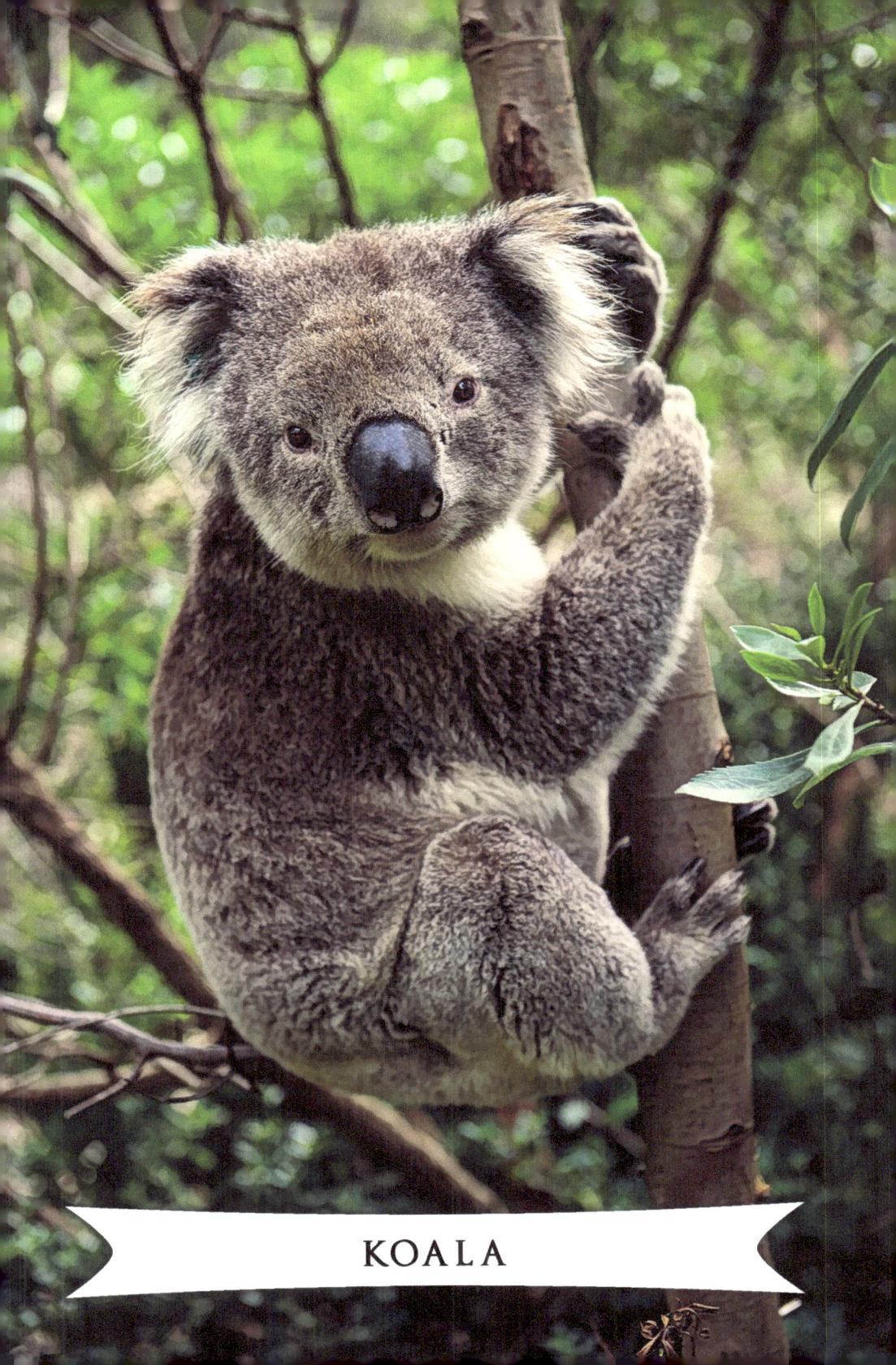
KOALA

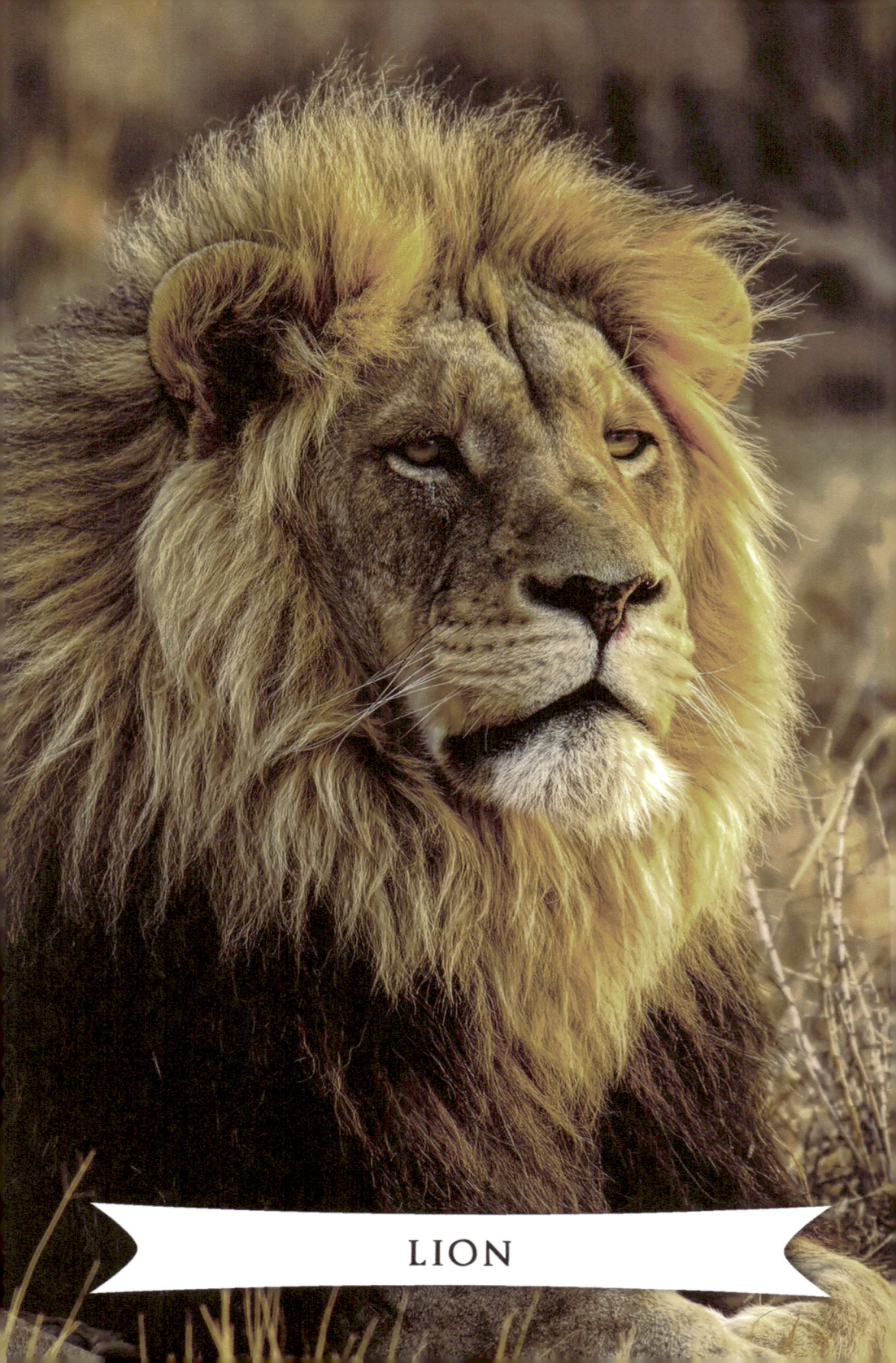

LION

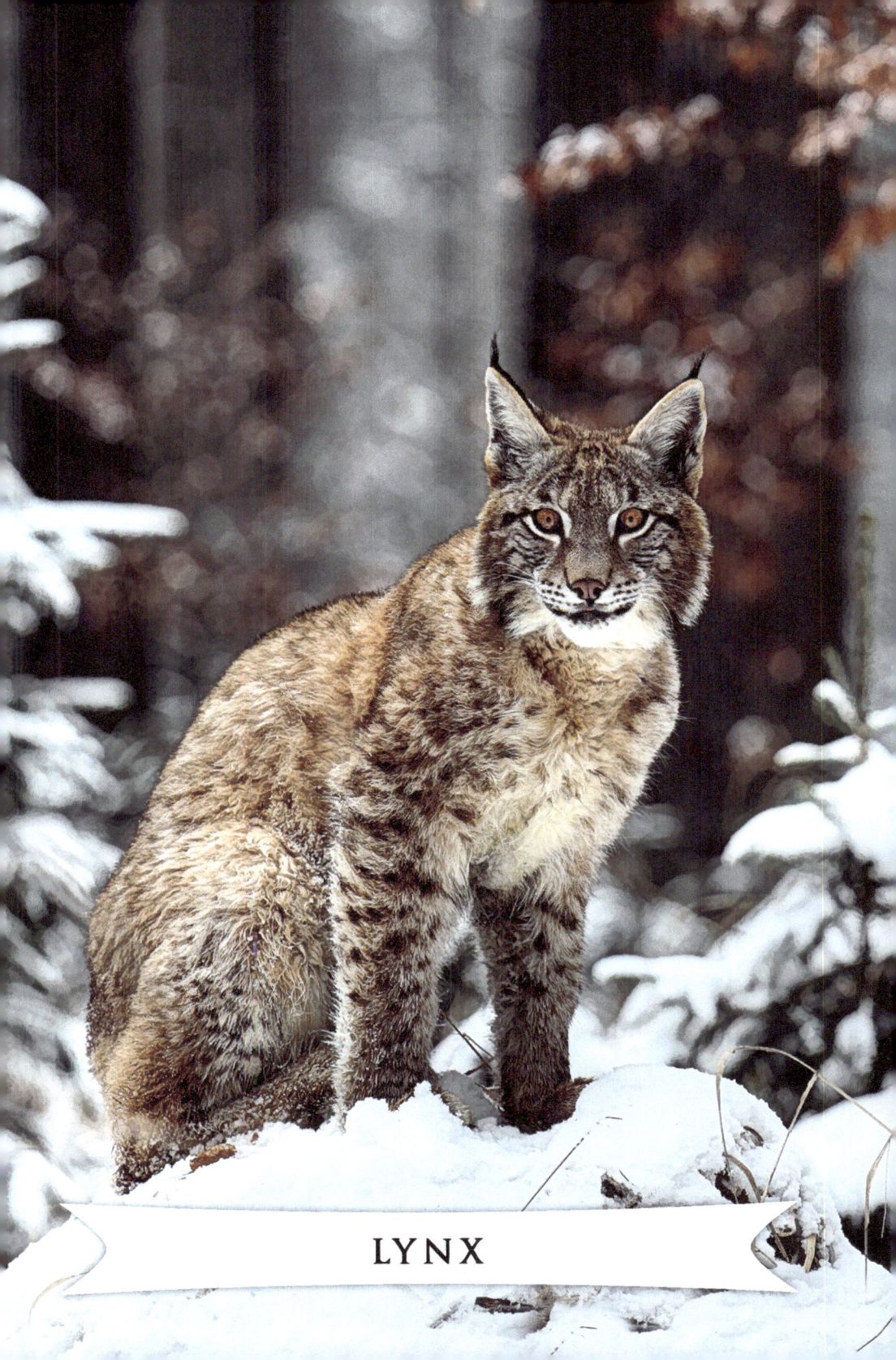

LYNX

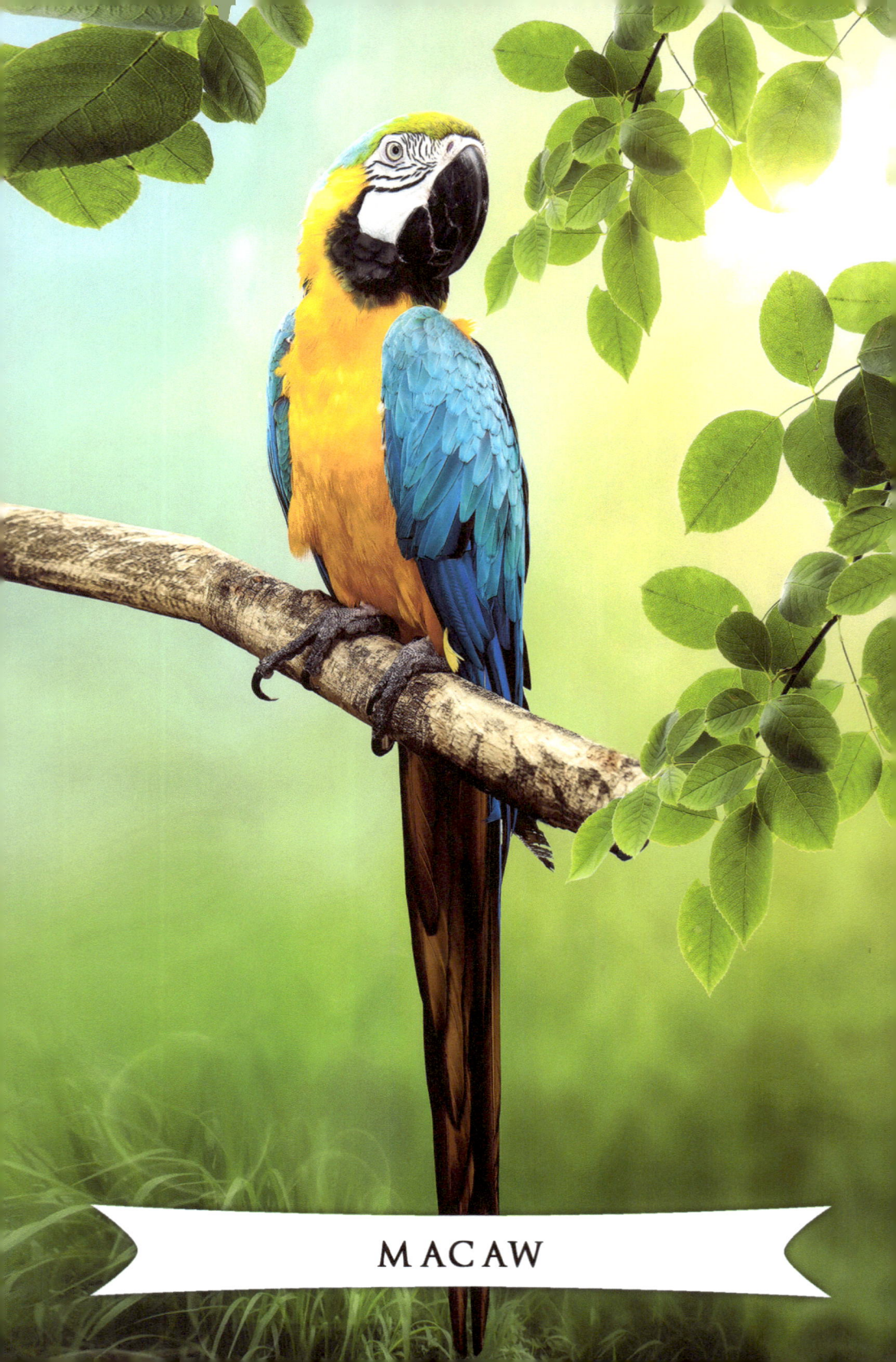

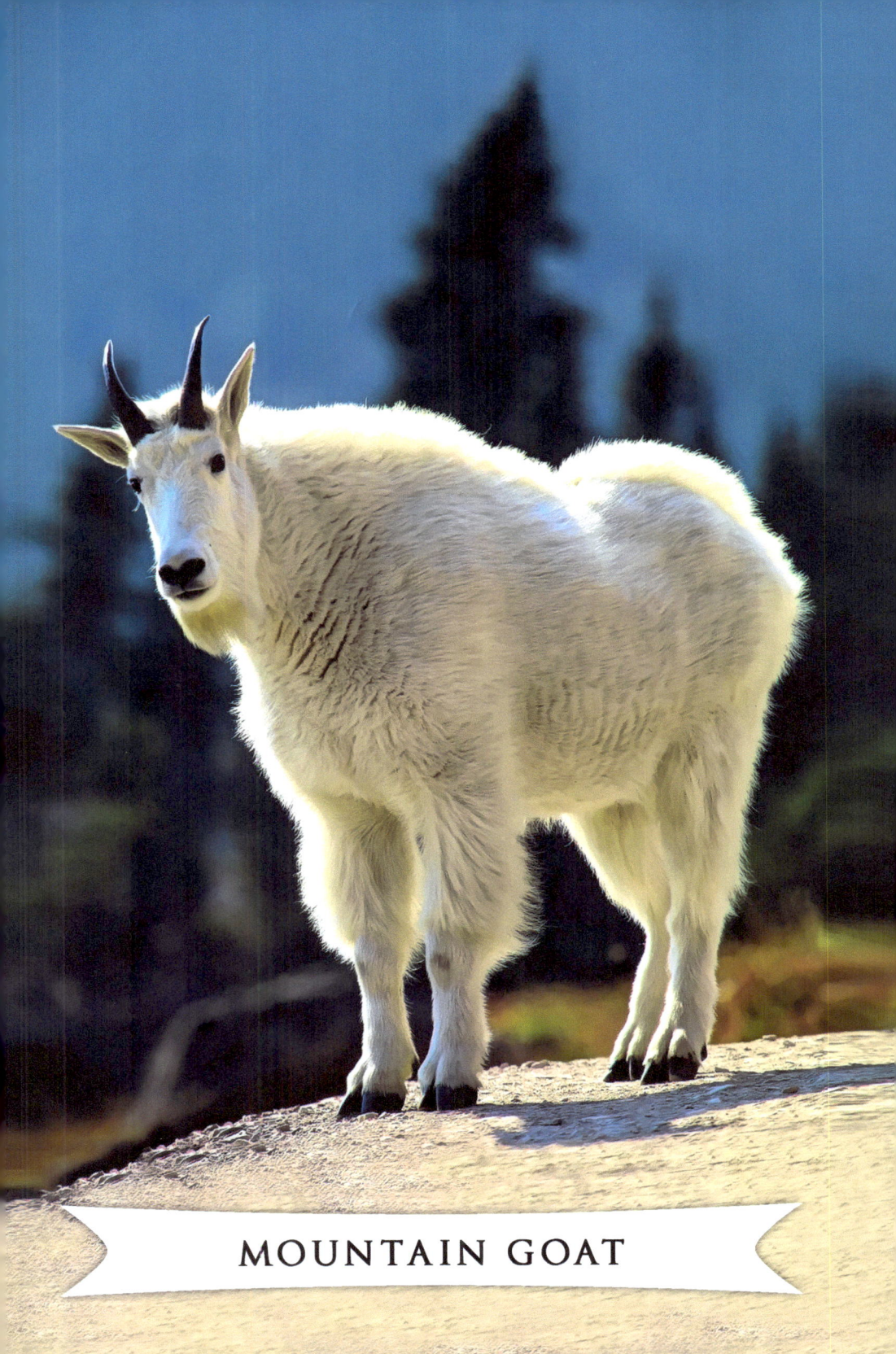

MOUNTAIN GOAT

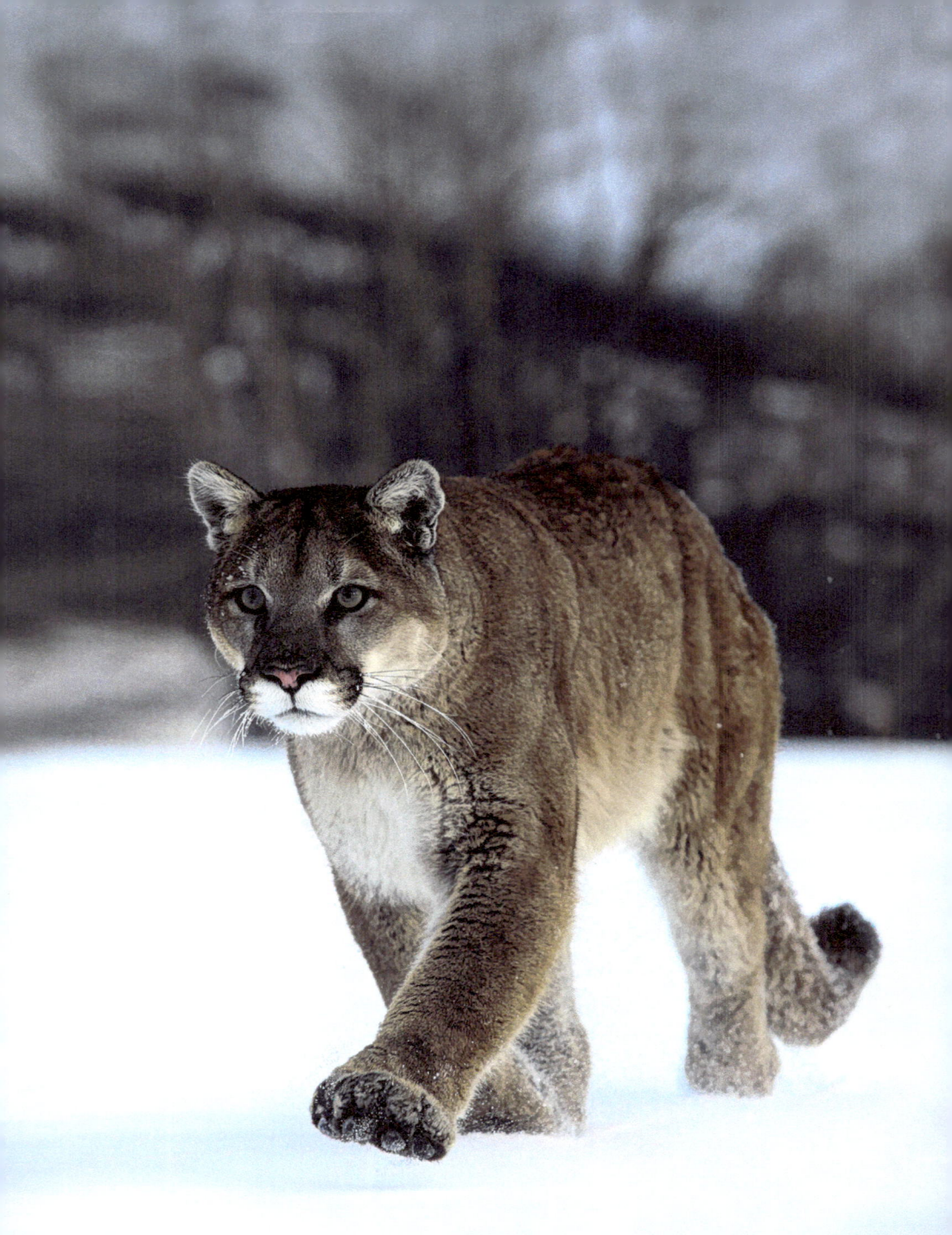

MOUNTAIN LION

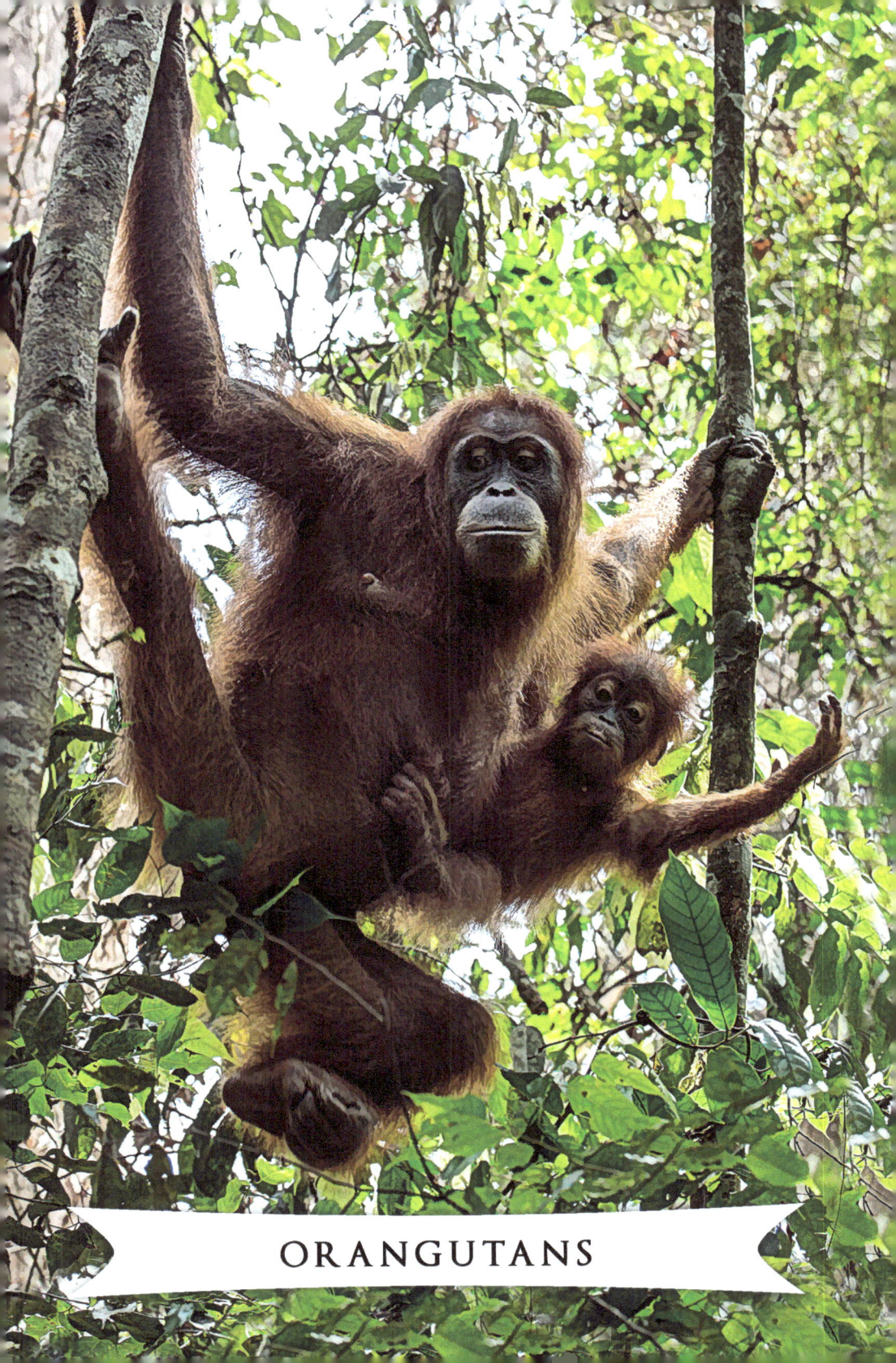

ORANGUTANS

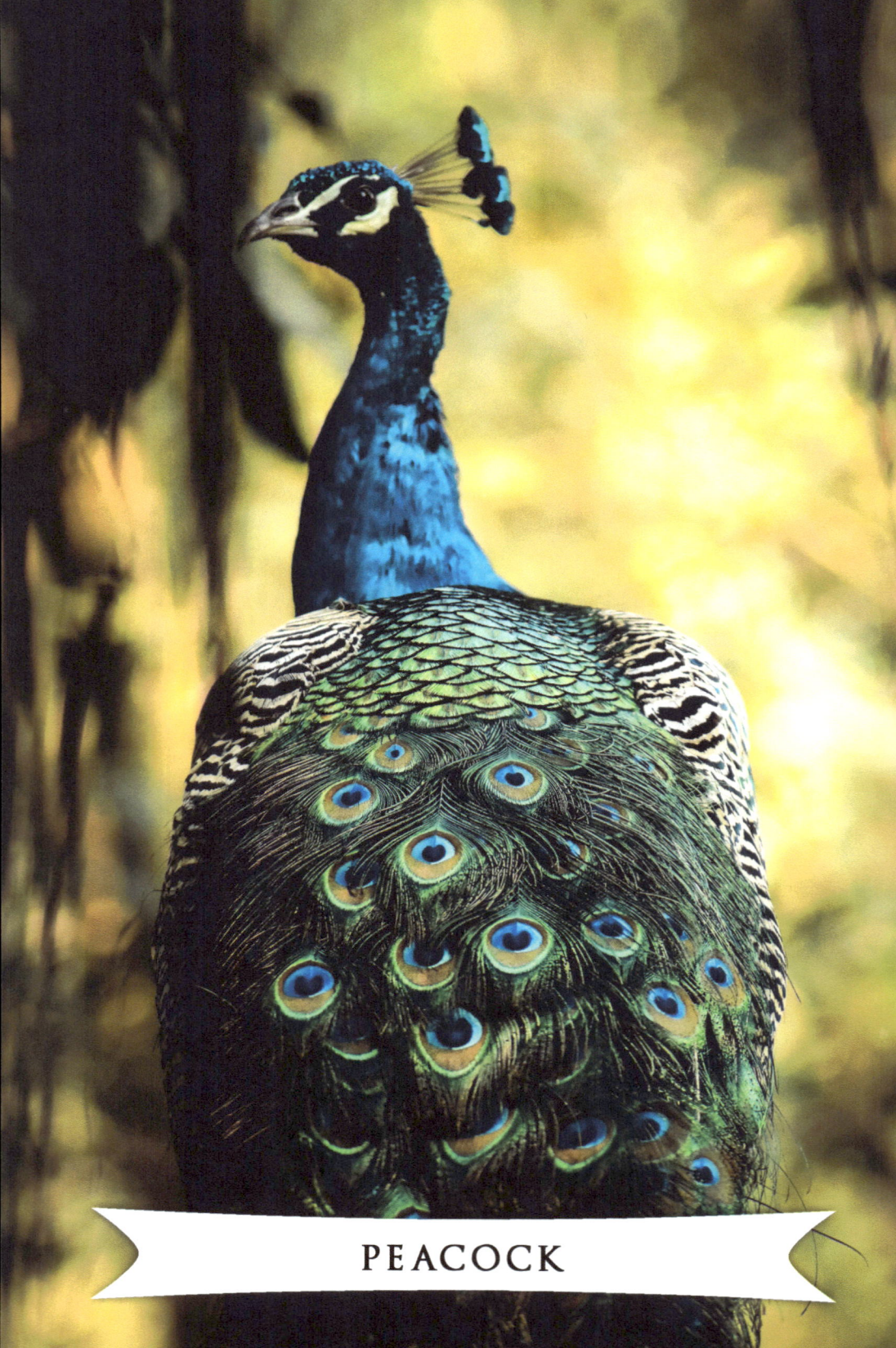

PEACOCK

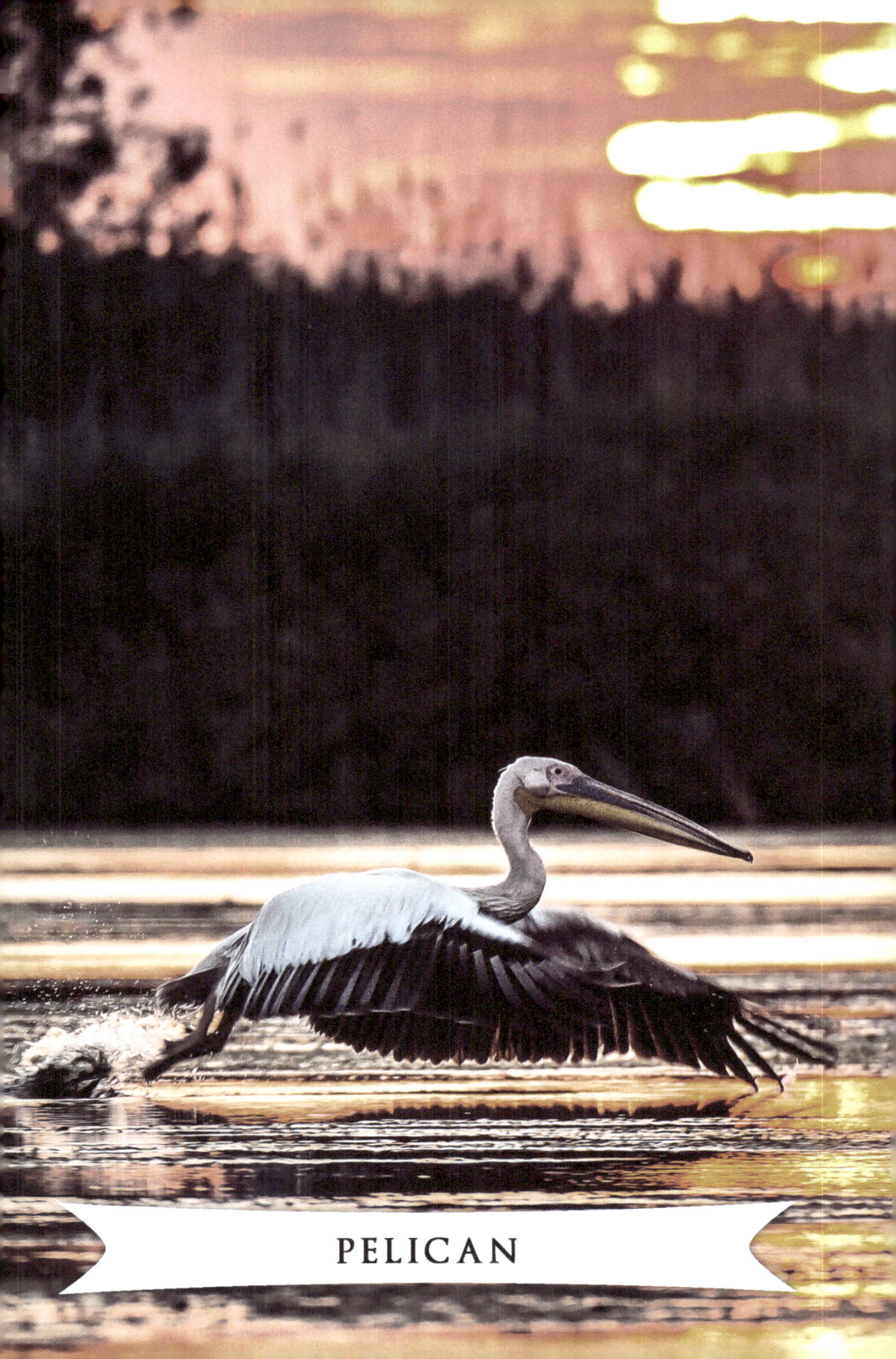
PELICAN

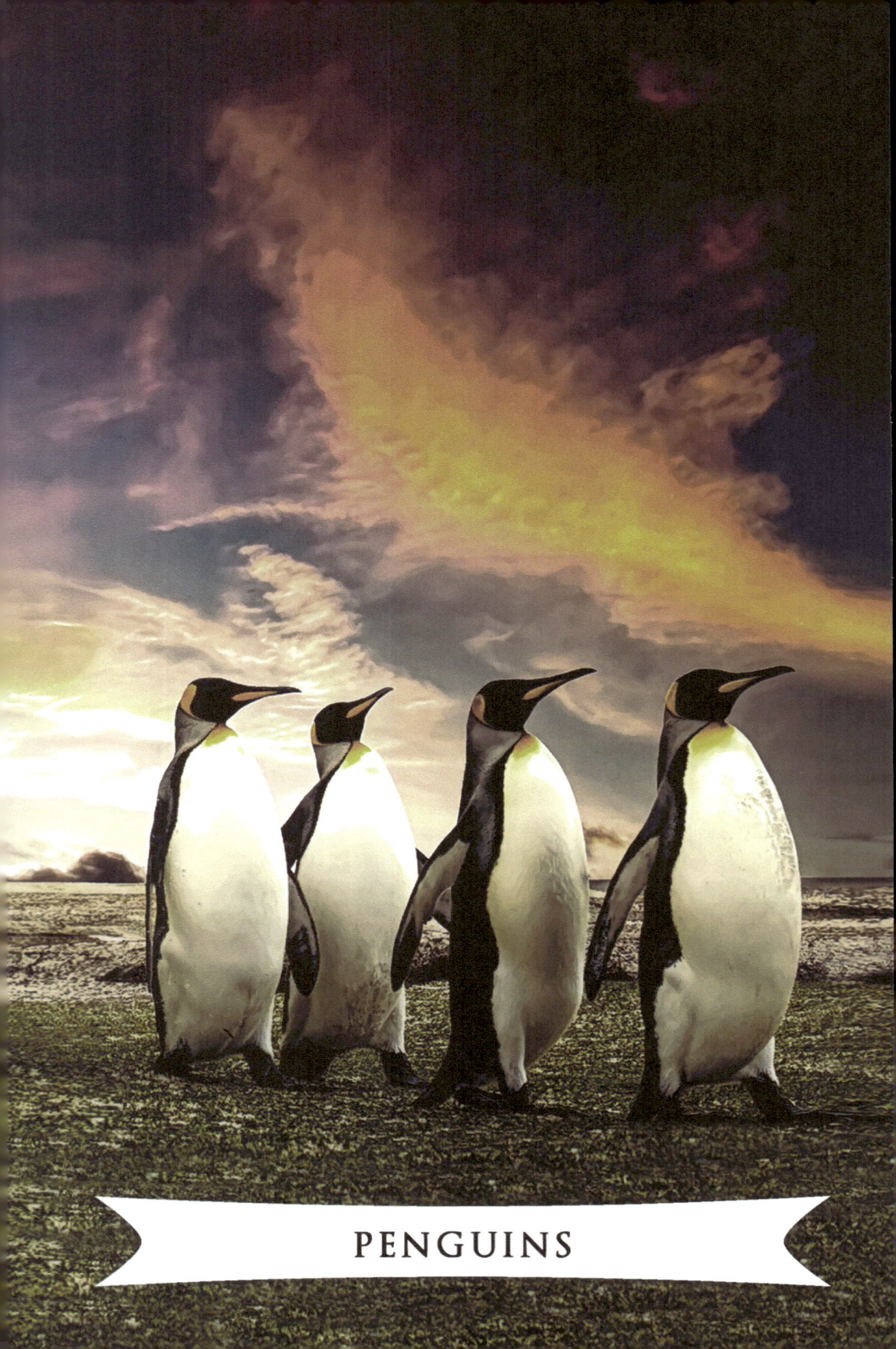

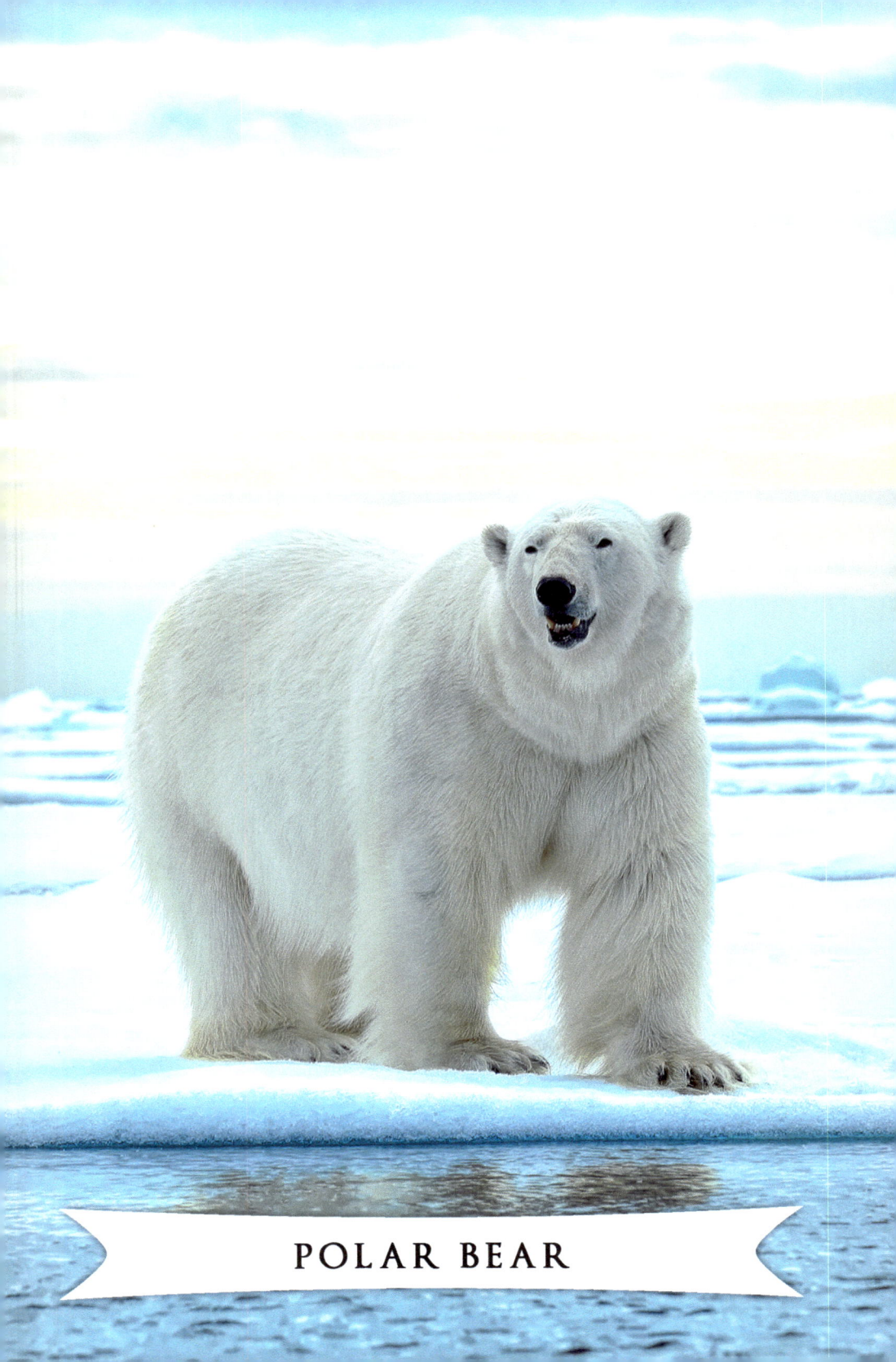

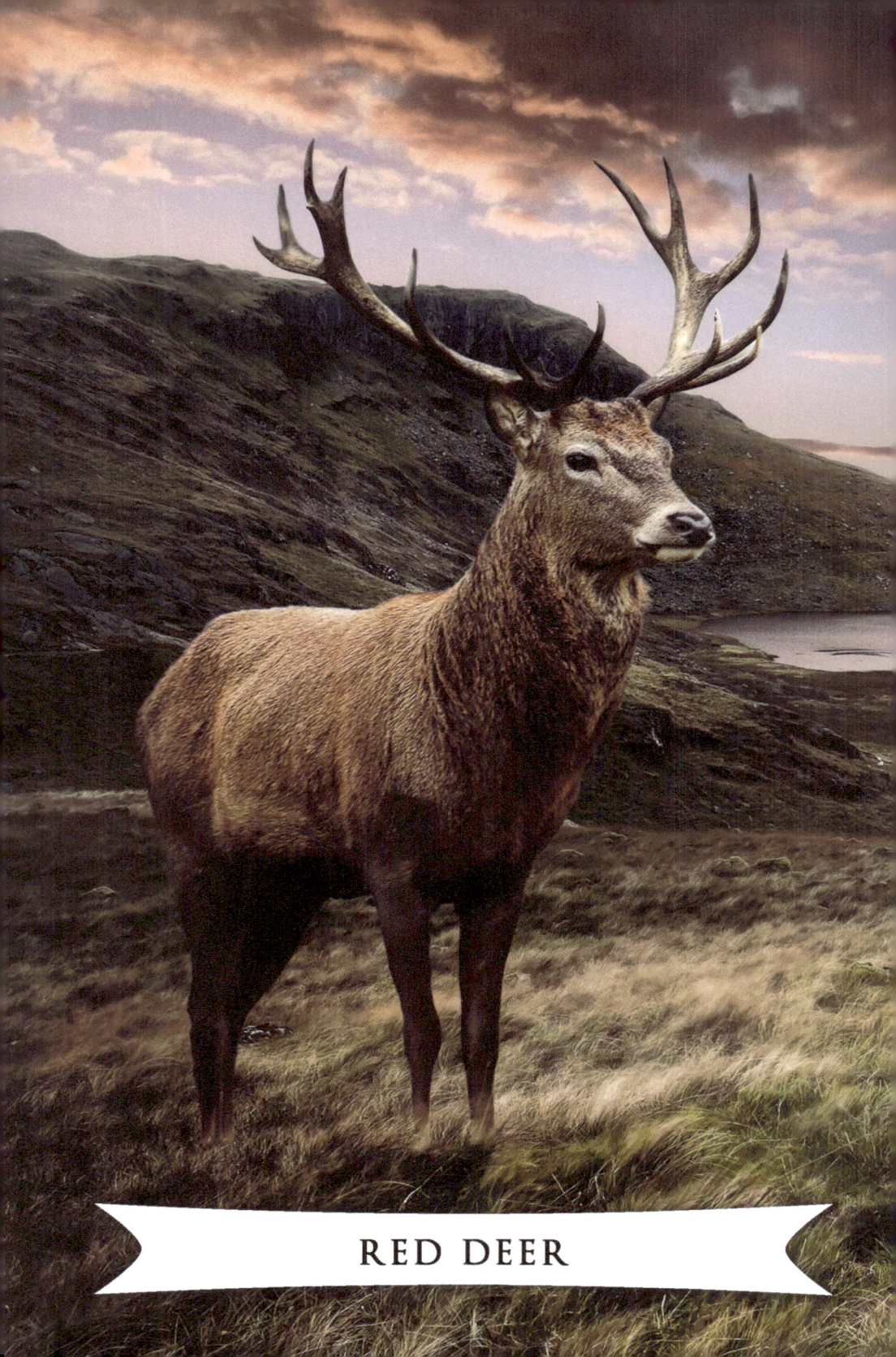

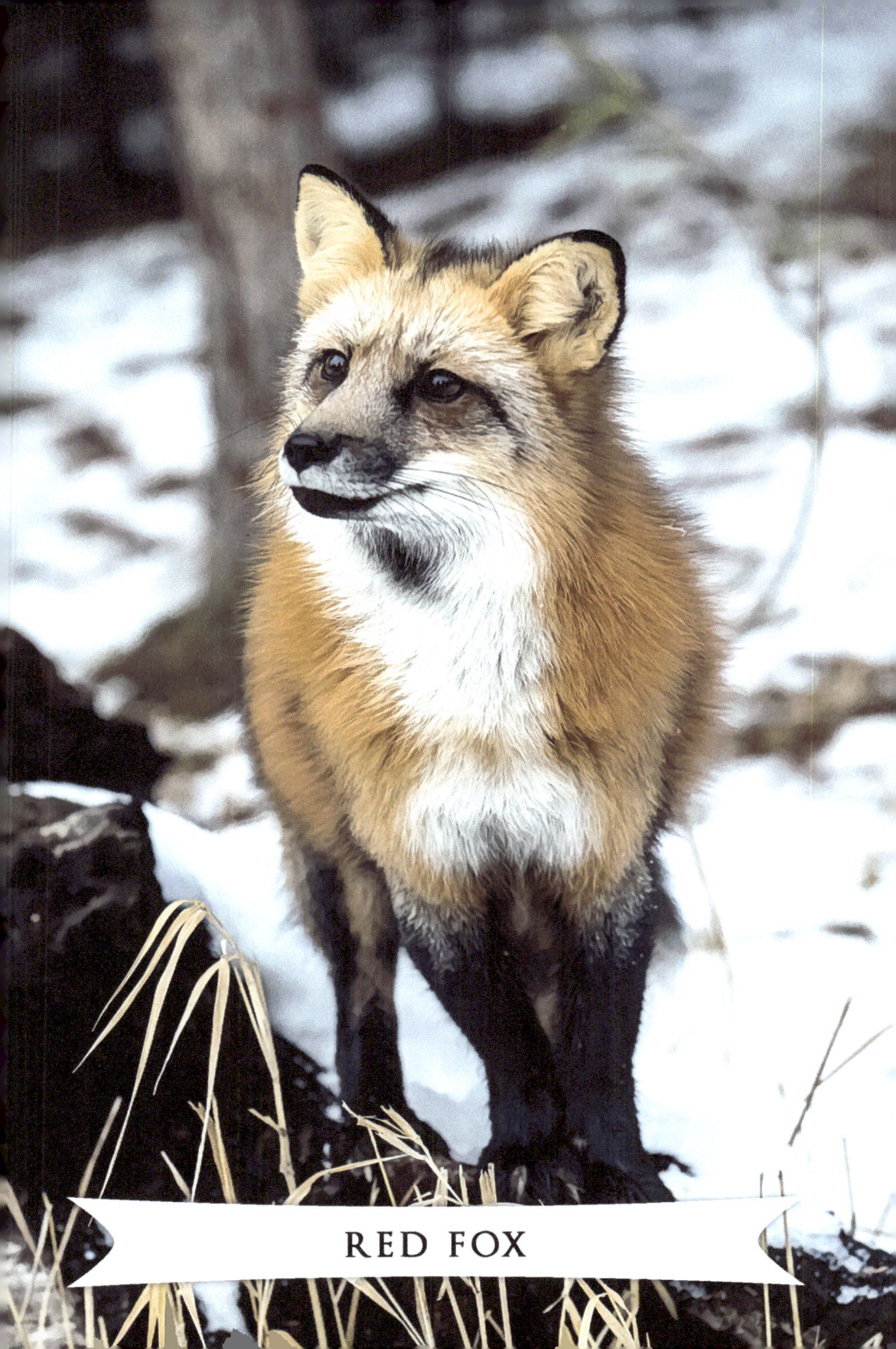

RED FOX

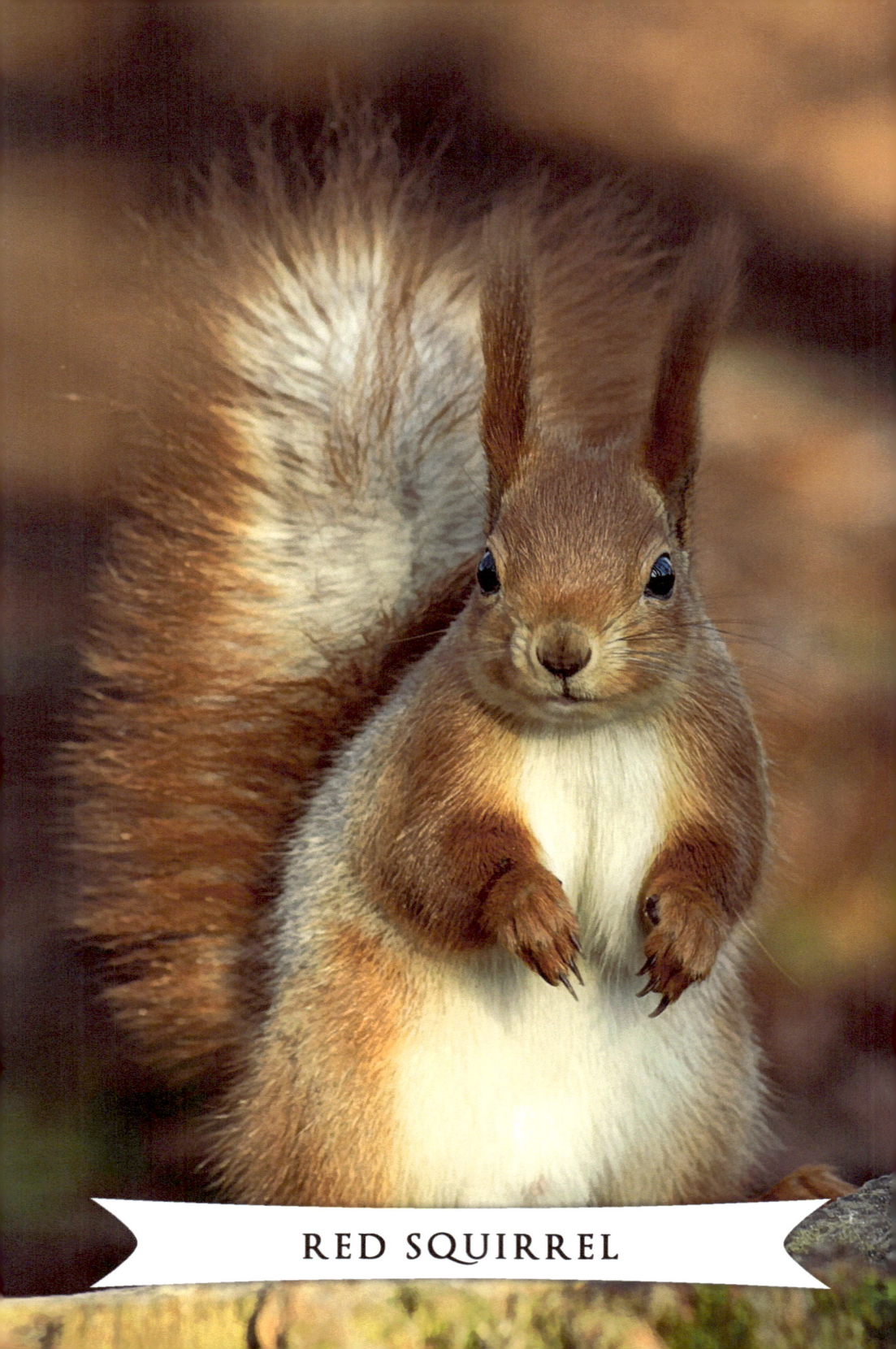

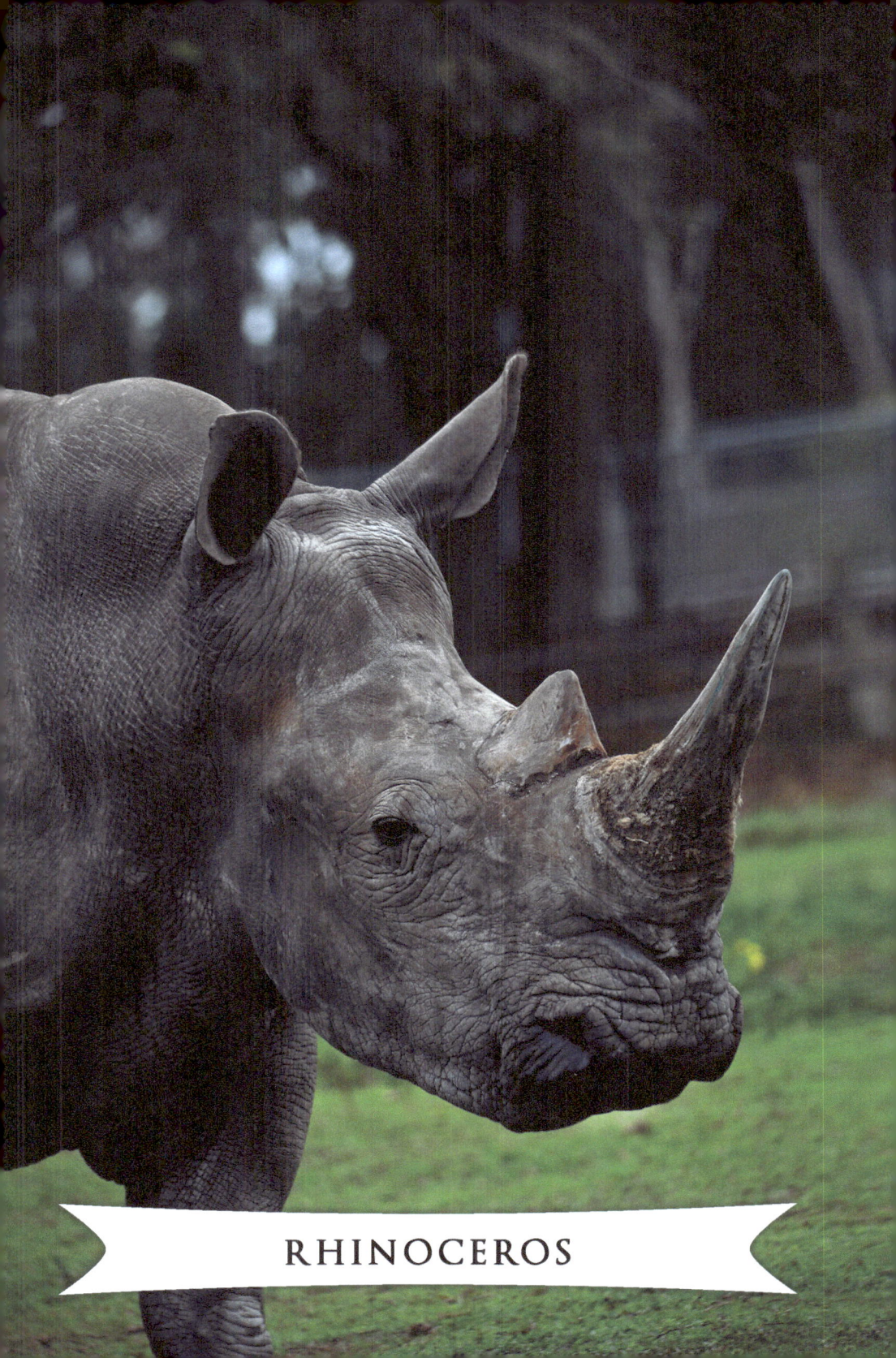

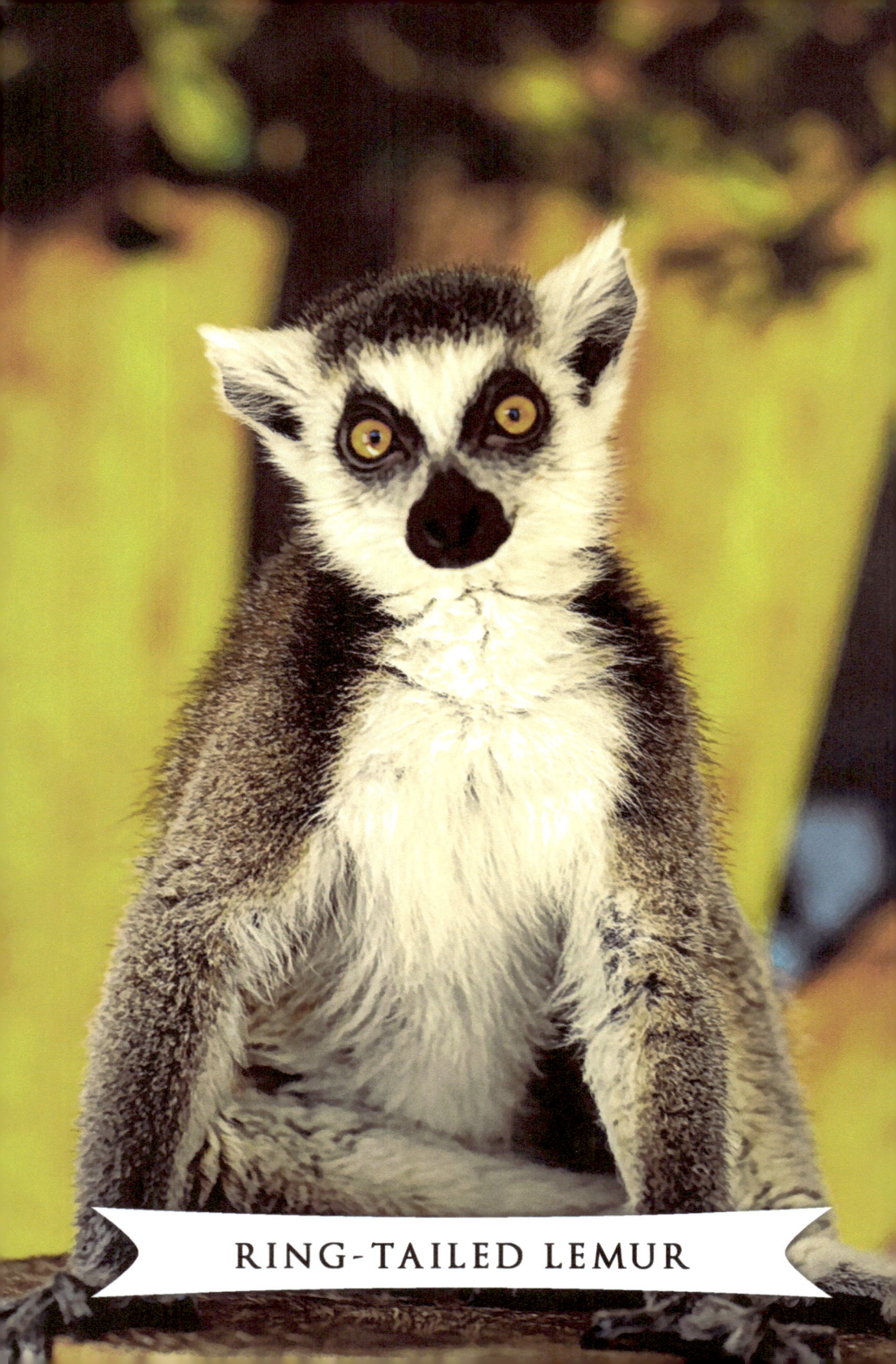
RING-TAILED LEMUR

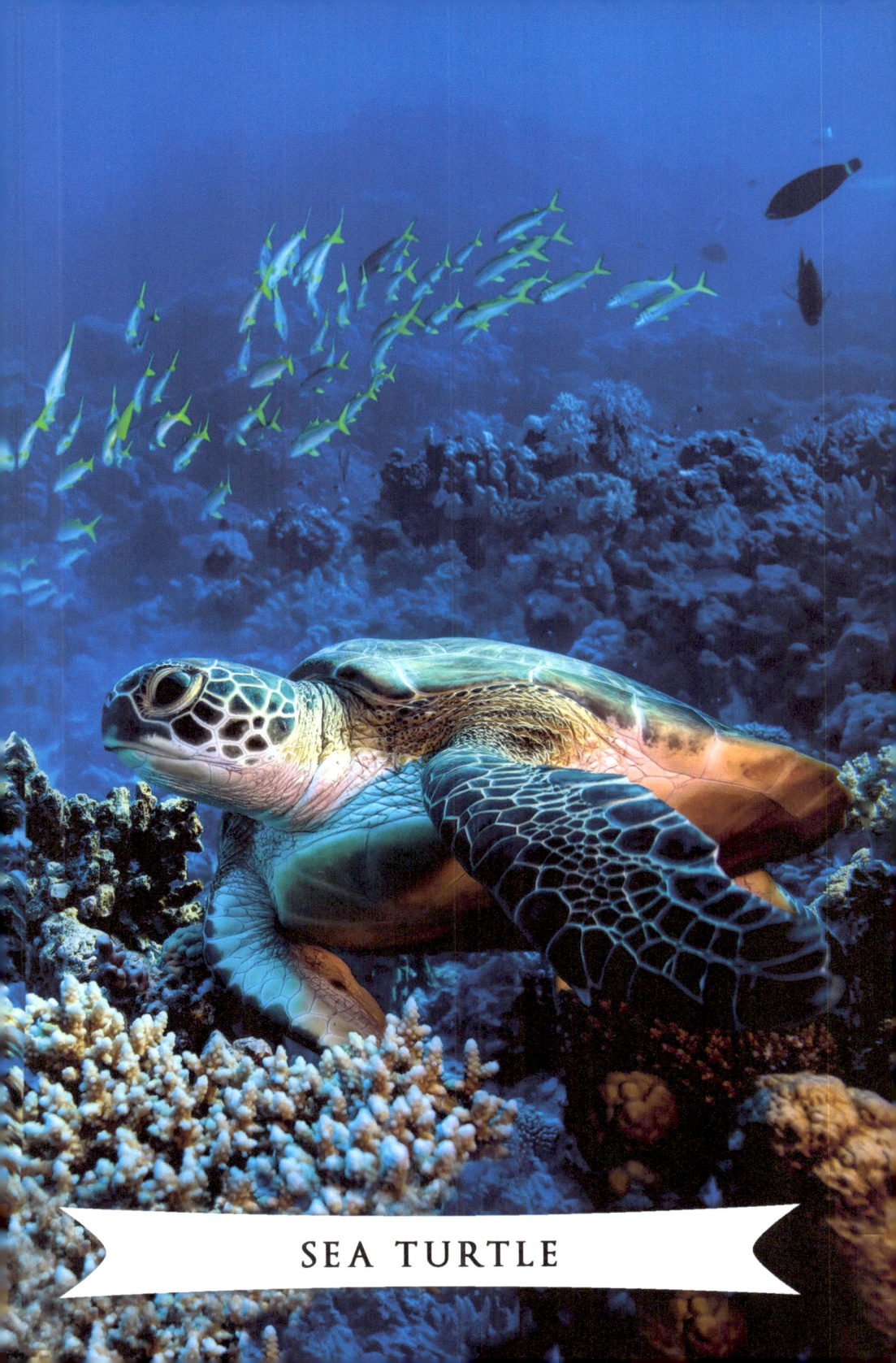

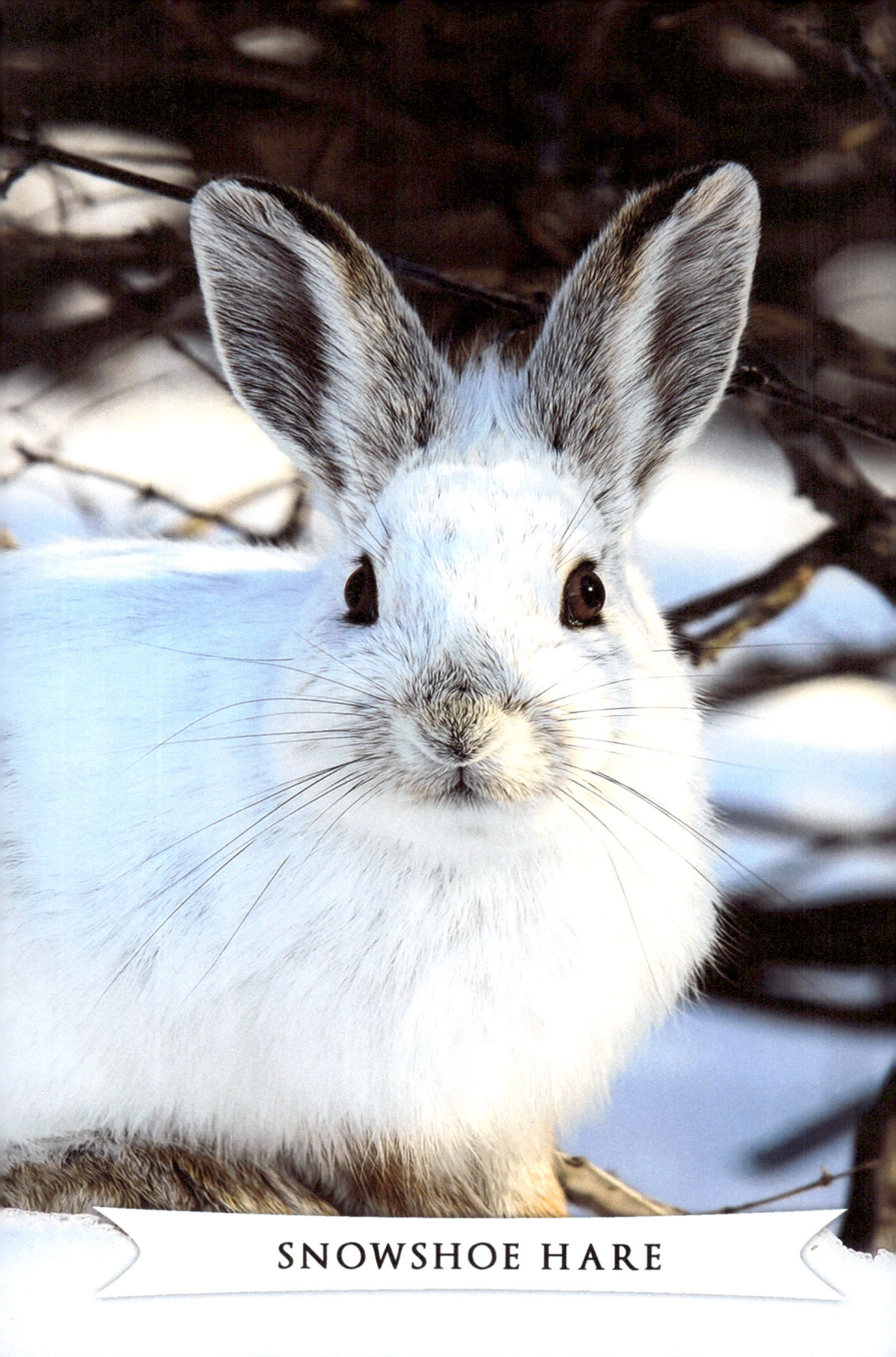
SNOWSHOE HARE

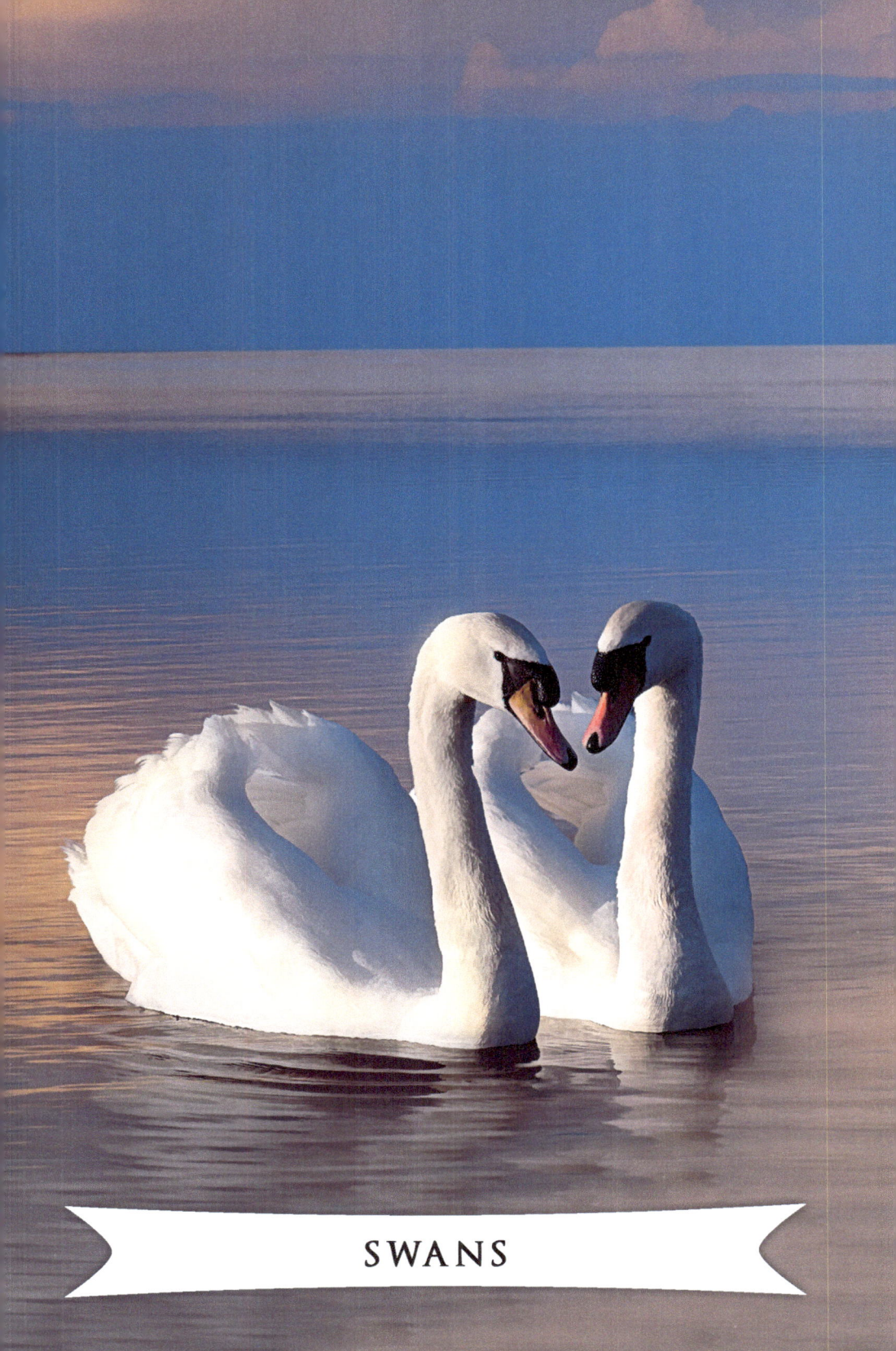
SWANS

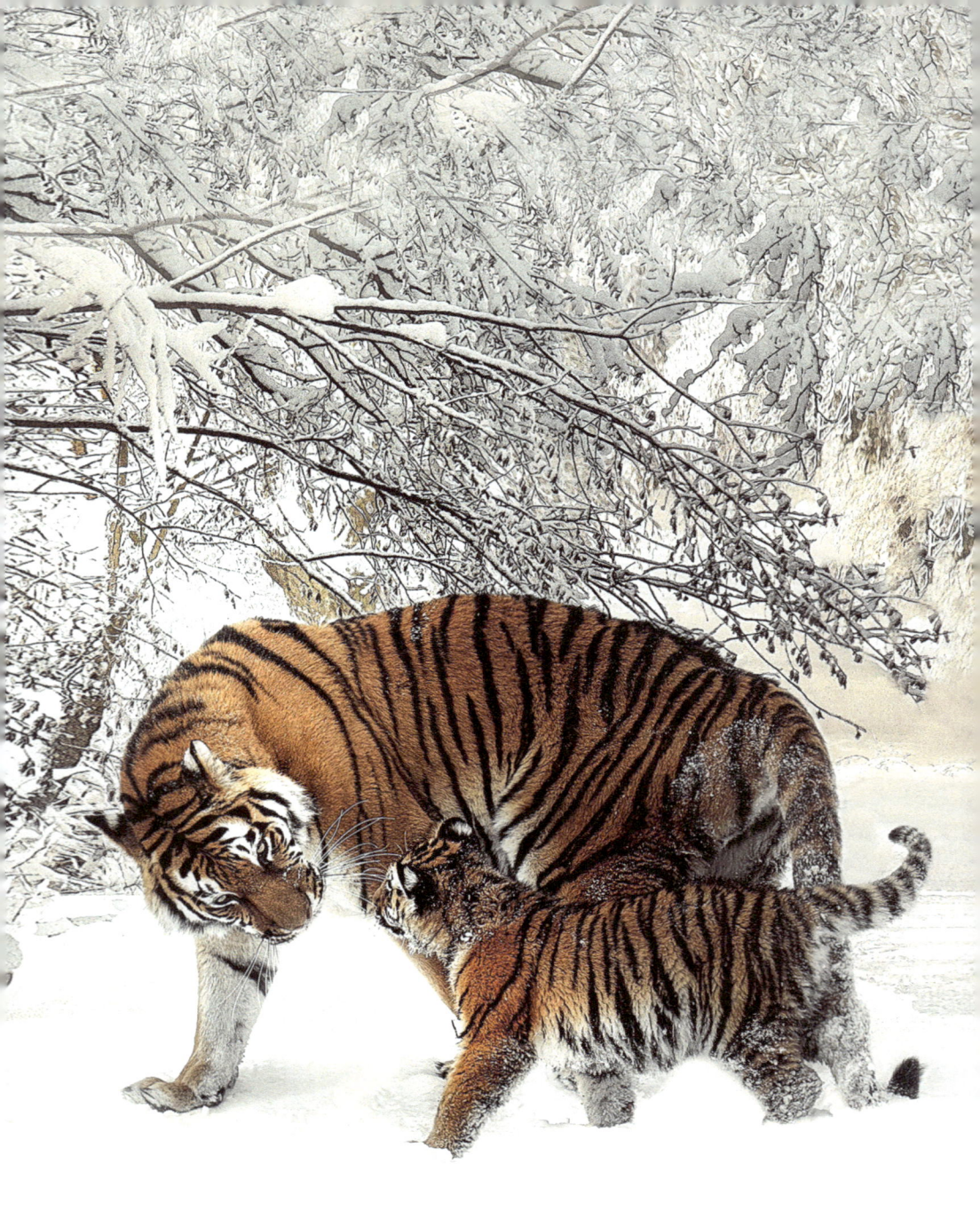

TIGERS

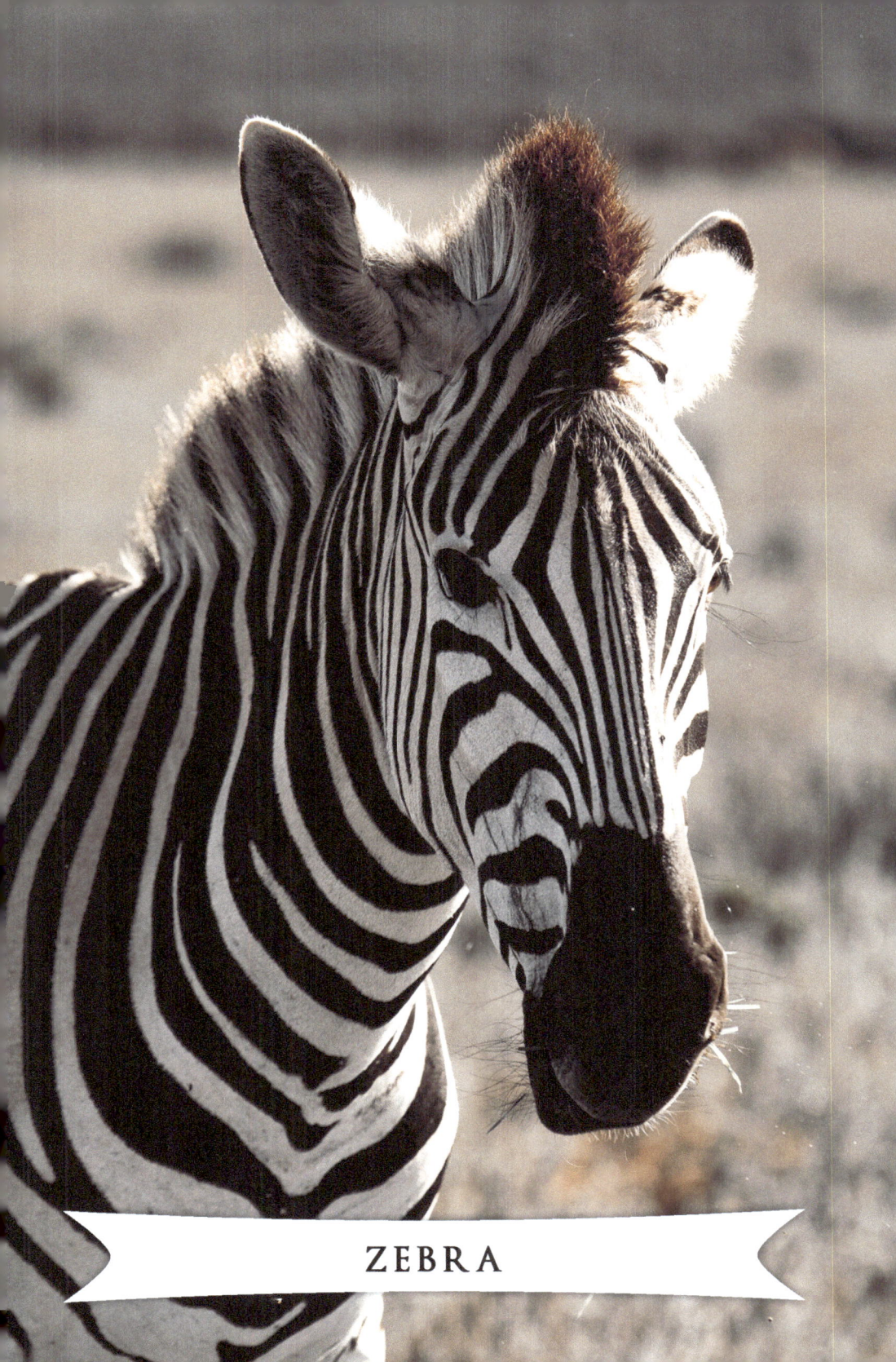

www.ingramcontent.com/pod-product-compliance
Lightning Source LLC
Chambersburg PA
CBHW040337220526
45473CB00009B/2712